I WAS ROBBED
OF MY DEATH!

Anne Beaudoin

I WAS ROBBED OF MY DEATH!

~ ~ ~

The End of a Collateral Damage

Translated from French
by Martine Beaudoin

Anne Marie Beaudoin Perron
Voces y Ecos del Corazón

Originally published as *On m'a volé ma mort!*

ISBN: 978-2-9816968-6-1

Québec (Québec), Canada
ambp.vocesyecosdelcorazon@gmail.com

Cover design: Anne Beaudoin
Front cover illustration: Anne Beaudoin
Revision: Diane Holmlund
Back cover photography: personal collection, July 2019

ISBN: 978-2-9819857-0-5
Legal deposit: 2022, *Bibliothèque et archives nationales du Québec*
Legal deposit: 2022, Library and Archives Canada

Print-on-demand publication

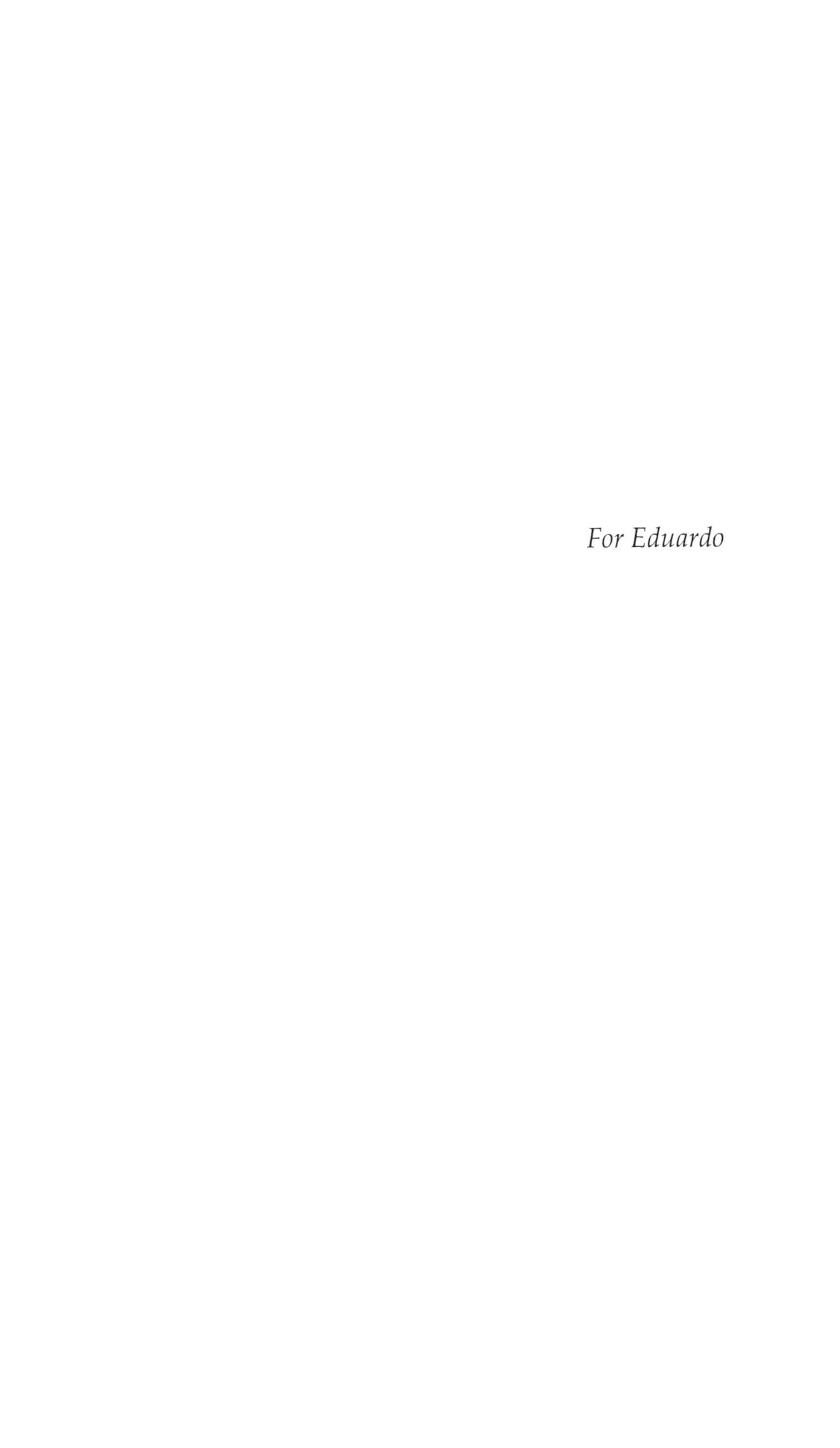

For Eduardo

Contents

Foreword xi

Introduction 1
The Last Moments 3
The Request 7
In Search of Information 11
Dialogue A 17
The Capacity for Discernment 19
Dialogue B 25
In Search of a Psychiatrist 31
Dialogue C 43
Preparing the Dossier 47
Dialogue D 57
The Letter to Peaceful Bridge 59
The Autobiographical Notice 63
The Last Times 67
A Transcendent Love 77
The Last Days 81

The End 101
At the End of His Struggle 113
About CPR 119
The Last Words 141

Notice: all the professionals mentioned in this story have fictitious names, except for Dr Georges L'Espérance and Dr Pierre Viens. Also fictitious are the following names: Growing Path, Peaceful Bridge and Lausterberg.

Foreword

When I entered the Faculty of Medicine in 1986, little did I know that my career would not follow the course I had imagined.

What was my ambition? I wanted to become a physician and take care of people. From my first year of study, when I met patients whose anamnesis I had to take, I felt deeply challenged by everything that I was beginning to touch. I was becoming aware of all the faces disease can take, of all the ramifications deriving from it, of all it reveals and can mean in sufferings and anxieties in someone's life. Would I be up to the task?

I did not doubt for long. With enthusiasm I threw myself in a never-ending apprenticeship and I became a physician. Happy to put myself at the service of others, I learned to care for them day after day, conscious of my limitations and of my vulnerability. Before the imposing reality of the life stories to which I was confronted, I always felt very small but never really powerless. Because I could always take care, support each patient and his/her parents as best as I could, being fully present and attentive to their particular needs. Whatever the circumstances were, I always tried to keep in mind the most important thing: the well-being of my patient.

I passionately loved my work as a pediatrician, as much in hospital as in first line clinic. I took up and enjoyed the everyday challenges with satisfaction; and I received, wholeheartedly, the small and great joys the children were giving me without knowing it. I also lived heartbreaking situations. One of them left me with indelible memories.

That day, I was on-call at the regional hospital where I was working. The day had been relatively peaceful and, after checking that all was well in the delivery ward, I had withdrawn to the room reserved for the on-call pediatrician. I was floating in a light sleep when my pager rang. I was needed at the operating room: an emergency cesarean! Acute fetal distress caused by uterine hypertonia. Full-term pregnancy, with no problem. The fetus was rapidly delivered from her mother's entrails, but it was already too late. The baby was dead, white as a sheet and unresponsive. So I did what was expected of me: I resuscitated her. If I hadn't done so, I would have risked paying a very high price. While the midwife was drying her and stimulating her, I aspirated her airway. Once intubated and ventilated, the baby regained some color and I took her to the Neonatology Unit. There I put her in an incubator and connected her to a mechanical ventilator. Then, I tried in vain to canalize the umbilical vessels. Tension was high. I had beside me the whole obstetrics-gynecology personnel assembled at the entrance of the Unit and anxiously looking through the crystal wall. I had the impression that everybody was expecting me to save the baby. As if it were obvious! Revolted by this bothering invasion, I asked that they would all go and let me work in peace.

"What have I done?" I told myself. I was in front of a stillborn baby that I was forcing to breathe with the help of a machine. If I persevered in my efforts, I would certainly end up canalizing the umbilical vessels, which would allow me to keep her on life support. But then, what? What future would this beautiful little girl with a tragic fate have? No. I was not going to fiercely work on her. Besides, the decision was not mine. I left the Unit to go converse with the father. I explained to him the critical state in which his daughter was. I couldn't make predictions, of course, but I could at least tell him frankly that the perspective was of the bleakest. Then, with a voice strangled by emotion but without any hesitation, he responded that he was absolutely incapable of having a "vegetable" as a daughter.

He refused to see the infant, but he insisted she be baptized. She was to be named Lucía. Thus, the hospital chaplain came to the Neonatology Unit in the middle of the night to celebrate the baptism of this poor creature whose life was ending before it had even begun. Gathered around the incubator where Lucía was lying still connected to the ventilator, the night nurse and her assistant and myself participated in the ceremony in a meditative way, very unusual for the place where we were. Before leaving the Unit, the chaplain asked me if I was certain of what I was doing, insinuating that it was perhaps worth trying again to bring the baby back into our world. His inopportune comment caught me off guard and I limited myself to respond succinctly. But, really, what was he imagining? That I was going to play the Supreme Being!?

After he left, I withdrew the respiratory assistance and remained by Lucía's side until her last breath, until her last heartbeat. The night nurse congratulated me for the way I had acted. She remarked that others would not have hesitated to work fiercely on the baby, which would have condemned her to an unbearable existence. I was glad she understood and gave me her support. After completing all the paperwork, exhausted, I returned to the room of the on-call pediatrician to recollect myself. I had just lived such a poignant event... I felt the need to be alone.

Two days later, after doing the maternity round, I went to visit Lucía's parents. Having had a cesarean, the mother was still hospitalized. I entered the room gently and I closed the door behind me. We talked in private... I think it was good for the three of us to come back on what had happened, without looking for a culprit. What touched me deeply is that they both thanked me, as much the mother as the father. They were grateful for the way I had intervened. I had reflected a lot about this traumatic night and I was blaming myself for some mishaps. But I had done my best in the circumstances, and they knew it. In listening to them telling me the painful moments they were living through, I felt my heart swollen with gratitude. Lucía's parents were welcoming me in the grief of their daughter, and I felt carried by the Infinite.

This story brings me to stress the incapacity for many doctors to face death. While it is difficult to accept the death of a child, this does not justify imposing on them treatments to prevent them from dying. Thinking that death is the worst thing that can happen makes us often lose sight of what is most important: the patient's well-being. Does not each human being, no matter how small they are, have their own fate? I mean by this that it is with humility and gentleness that we penetrate someone's sacred universe. It is not death that is unacceptable, but the fact of intervening by all means to prevent it from happening, to the point of creating inhuman and meaningless life situations. If the natural course of things was respected, the whole world would feel a lot better. As physicians, we do not have the obligation to prolong people's lives whatever it costs. Our mission is simply to take care of our patients with respect for their person.

For my part, I did not work as a pediatrician as long as I would have liked. The excessive interventionism characterizing today's medicine has had catastrophic consequences in the life of my son Eduardo and, by the same token, in mine. The day came where I chose to abandon my career in order to follow him until the end. My commitment toward him has been total and, today, by means of this book, it is with a double voice I bear witness: the voice of the mother, of course, but also the voice of the physician.

Anne Beaudoin

Introduction

This little work is part of the promise I made my son Eduardo before his passing: I committed myself to bear witness in his name, to go to the end of his mission, to exhaust all of my resources in order to make his story known to the world.

Dead at the age of six and brutally resuscitated, therefore condemned to live a terrible calvary, he did not understand why this had been done to him. Those who have read our book *Why was I resuscitated?* know that, in spite of all the obstacles that rose up before us, we journeyed together day after day, courageously, during endless years, seeking without respite the best way to live with so many limitations...

This book is the last chapter of a life filled with sufferings, frustrations and humiliations of all kinds, repeated invariably each day, the last chapter of a life that was not his and that he did not want anymore.

Not only was Eduardo unafraid of death, but he said that "death is the goal of life." And he was determined to reclaim his death.

Eduardo: a wonderful, formidable and admirable being who impressed me every day of our life together. Dynamic, energetic, intrepid and eager to experience life, he did not support any longer to be imprisoned and deprived of everything.

Victim of a reductionist and utilitarian medicine and of a health system where, unfortunately, protocols and productivity objectives prevail over the respect of the person, Eduardo went to die where he was welcomed in his suffering, the suffering of a mutilated being.

Here is, in the following pages, the story of his liberation process.

The Last Moments

The day awaited with so much intensity and hope has arrived at last.

The room where we are is ample and luminous. We breathe peacefulness in spite of the immensity of what is about to happen. There is Dr Gisela Kosch, her assistant in the procedure and a witness. And of course, I am there also, always inhabited by an anguish that compresses my heart.

Eduardo is settled on the adjustable bed, in a semi-reclined position. He is serene, without any apprehension, radiating with determination, content that this moment be now before him. His left arm is connected to an IV line hooked to a support beside the bed. Everything is ready. Gisela asks him four questions:

"What is your name?"

"Eduardo García Beaudoin."

"When were you born?"

"On August 6, 1996."

"On August 8, 1996?"

"On August 6."

"On August 6, 1996. Very well, very well. Eduardo, why have you come here?"

"To ask for medical aid in dying."

"To ask for medical aid in dying. Because you cannot [...] and you have this tetraplegia bothering you a lot, no? Eduardo, I put a drip line. Do you know what will happen if you open the line now?"

"Die."

"Die, you are going to die."

"Mhmm."

"Yes, yes. So, Eduardo, if what you most want is to die, you may open now."

Eduardo starts to manipulate the tubing.

"I know it is very, very difficult for you. You take your time."

I look at him and I watch him make considerable efforts to hold well the tubing. I hear him moan a little seeing he cannot do it.

"Eduardo, if you want you can sit," says Gisela.

So Eduardo straightens up on the bed. With his left hand, wrist locked in a complete flexion, he holds the tubing the best he can, while with his right index and thumb, he manipulates with difficulty the opening mechanism of the drip line, a small wheel he must push upward. It is a crucial moment, a long awaited moment, another wrestling moment, a moment filled with tension and hope... From where I stand, behind Gisela and her assistant (who is filming), I am unable to see his hands and to observe the progress of his efforts; but, suddenly, I perceive his satisfied countenance looking upward, toward the small transparent bag containing the lethal medication that starts flowing in him and that is going to give him back his death. And I understand he has succeeded in opening the perfusion. Deliverance! At last! He is free. He is soaring in Eternity...

The Request

It was the beginning of the year 2018, the end of February or beginning of March. Eduardo was eating his supper. I was already finished and, as usual, I had turned on the TV to listen to *MétéoMédia*. Before switching to Chanel 21, we had time to hear the news of the moment about medical aid in dying (MAID). It was an update on the last developments concerning the proceedings undertaken by Mrs Nicole Gladu and Mr Jean Truchon to contest the constitutionality of the federal and provincial laws about medical aid in dying.

Eduardo caught the news in its entirety and declared, "Me, I want it now, the medical aid in dying." I turned off the TV on the spot. I sat with him at the table again and I asked him to repeat what he had just said.

"Me, I want it now, the medical aid in dying."

I could see he was serious and he knew perfectly what he was saying. I was also realizing, without being fully aware of it at the time, that I no longer needed to rack my brain and my soul—a real torture!—to try to make him understand there was no end to his predicament, there was no hope for improvement. He had understood this by himself and, with the determination I knew to be his, he was already expressing his desire without faltering.

On that day an extensive ground work started for us, multiple exchanges in depth and months of meticulous endeavors, which he called his "project." I preferred speaking of it as his liberation process.

In our book, published in October 2017 in its original version (Spanish) and whose French translation was well on its way the day he expressed his request for MAID, I relate how he has set for himself the goal to walk again and that he is convinced he can achieve it. Therefore, I was asking myself, what had happened between October 2017 and now? I had noticed he had become sombre. He was maintaining his energy level and was continuing to go to the PEPS (Laval University's sports and physical education pavilion) with the same frequency and the same diligence. He was working on his internet puzzles and his colorings with the same interest and the same concentration. He had even kept his sense of humour, joking about everything and laughing out loud in watching *Caméra Café*, *Shin Chan* or *The Simpsons*; but the light that had always brightened his eyes was gone. His gaze was in the dark.

He told me that he could not take anymore being in a wheelchair, that he was before an insuperable wall, that he was suffering in his wounded soul, that he wanted to go to heaven... He felt demolished. If he could not walk again, he did not want to stay in this world.

In Search of Information

Eduardo had made a decision and he was relying on me to bring it into reality. I welcomed with an open heart the task he was entrusting me with, while perceiving in the depth of myself that, according to his will, a long and painful combat was beginning.

We talked a lot. We talked every day, I think. About his decision, his situation, about everything he had lived through and was continuing to live, about what he wanted and what he did not want. I asked him a multitude of questions to help him verbalize what for him did not need explaining. I absolutely needed him to make explicit in his own words where he was on the road of his existence, the view he had on the life he was living, what he felt at the core of himself, what his needs were and what he yearned for.

All this was not easy because Eduardo was a man of a few words. Moreover, for him everything was clear. His decision made sense to him, implacable logic. Why did others not see it? Why did others not understand it? Why did he have to prove anything? I explained and repeated to him as many times as needed that there was no choice, that things must be done according to the law. To maximize the chances for his "project" to succeed, everything ought to be in order, in the smallest details. And so as the time was passing and weighing on us, our conversations continued until the end.

Our life was following its habitual course, but from one day to the next my days became saturated by a new activity: I started to navigate the internet, seeking information on medical aid in dying. Every day, while Eduardo was killing time in his diverse interactions with the computer, I was using the iPad and I was searching... I must say it is with a feeling of bitterness—almost of revolt—that I threw myself into my research since, on account of the very restrictive criteria of the Canadian and Québec laws, Eduardo was not eligible to access medical aid in dying in his country. Indeed, in spite of the *Carter* decision of February 2015—in which the Supreme Court of Canada rules that "legislation prohibiting assisted dying infringes the right to life, liberty and security of the person under section 7 of the Canadian Charter of Rights and Freedoms"—, the Quebecer and Canadian lawmakers had not properly fulfilled their task. In Québec, we continued to restrict MAID to people who are at the end of life, while refusing categorically to adjust the provincial law to its federal counterpart; and in Canada, the law modifying the Criminal Code, that became effective in July 2016, was limiting MAID to people whose natural death has become reasonably foreseeable, a vague and rather ludicrous concept, let us say it, considering the high tech society in which we live. Eduardo had died on November 20, 2002, but he had been resuscitated... he was in an unbearable situation and he was suffering in an unspeakable manner, but he was no longer at the end of life. Therefore we had to look elsewhere.

At the time of addressing his request, because our two laws were being contested, the debates surrounding MAID had started again and the media, of course, were echoing them. I was remembering bitterly the legislative works preceding the adoption of the federal law. We had heard things like "It is difficult to verify if the sufferings of someone are intolerable," "We must allow a sufficient time period for reflection (10 days!) between the request for MAID and its administration to make sure the person has well considered the issue," or "It is necessary for the person to be able to consent up to the last moment before administering MAID." What a lack of humanity!

With the discussions on the subject resuming, I was once more outraged by the many opinions television and the internet were bringing to me. What should we think, for example, when our leaders keep repeating, without being able to prove it, that the criterion of death reasonably foreseeable has been added to protect vulnerable people? To protect them from what? From their freedom of choice? And in Québec, we were arguing, among other things, that MAID could not be considered as a treatment for people who are not at the end of life. Really? I believe the law-makers would have needed to spend, if only a short week end, imprisoned in a humiliating indignity and being prey to intolerable suffering in order to understand the realities of people requesting MAID.

However, the Supreme Court had been very clear in the *Carter* decision and did not invoke the proximity of natural death but rather the respect of the will of the person and the alleviation of their suffering. Why was this discriminatory factor introduced into the law? Did the people who had legislated know what they were talking about? They evidently had not understood what the Supreme Court had asked them or they had simply decided not to comply. Or maybe it was just about politics after all? Whatever it is, the criteria of "death reasonably foreseeable" and of "end of life" were being contested before the Superior Court of Québec, and we had no hope that the matter would be settled positively in an acceptable time frame.

But the reality here was not about to discourage me. I was going to find an exit door for Eduardo. I read and watched a lot of documents: articles, interviews, testimonies, reports, essays, official texts... I familiarized myself with what is happening in the world and with the diverse organizations working for the right to die with dignity. I was glad to realize the existence of all these groups of people defending a right as fundamental as this.

And so, I eventually found myself on the website Dignitas – To live with dignity – To die with dignity, a Swiss organization I had vaguely heard of before. In surveying the site, I discovered plenty of things that led me to plenty of others. I found the testimony of a Québec woman, professor and researcher, who voluntarily put an end to her life in 2017 and who denounces the cowardliness of our elected officials and the doctors' hypocrisy on the matter of MAID. I had the opportunity to read the excerpt of an essay written by a German specialist on medical ethics who considers that fighting against diseases is not an end in itself, that the task of medicine is to alleviate the suffering of human beings and that this task must always be accomplished with respect for patient self-determination. He considers that when the basis for medical ethics is "the alleviation of suffering and respect of self-determination, it seems evident it is completely compatible with assisted suicide." That meets my view: doctors must take care of their patients, always respecting who they are and what is important to them. I firmly believe that respect for the person must be at the heart of medical action. Yes, if we respect the person, the so-called ethical conflicts—which are nothing more than mind constructs—disappear automatically.

In short, I had found Dignitas, a not-for-profit organization whose activities are based on the freedom of choice, the respect for human dignity throughout life (that is to say until death) and the right to self-determination for everyone. Working mainly in the field of palliative care and suicide attempt prevention, it offers to its members, among others, end-of-life advice and support, as well as assisted dying. This help is extended to members who are not Swiss citizens. There are specific conditions to be fulfilled to receive the assisted suicide aid: to be a member of Dignitas, to be of sound judgement and to possess a minimum level of physical mobility. Furthermore, since the participation of a Swiss physician is necessary, the member must suffer from either a diagnosed terminal illness, an unendurable incapacitating disability, unbearable and uncontrollable pain, or from a combination of the three. Therefore Eduardo was admissible!

Now the time had come to knock at Dignitas door. In a first email prepared with care, I presented Eduardo's case in a clear and concise manner, mentioning that here, MAID was exclusively reserved for people at the end of life—but they certainly knew that. Since I had already collected much information from their website, I asked them a list of very specific questions in order to be able to adequately prepare ourselves and to plan the process in a realistic way. They answered me promptly sending me three PDF documents: a form for joining the organization and two information pamphlets, one about their providing assisted suicide and the other explaining how Dignitas functions and what are its philosophical principles. After reading everything attentively, I felt ready to put myself to work, to begin the task that would lead to my son's liberation; but there was an issue still seriously bothering me... Would the fact that Eduardo was under guardianship constitute an obstacle for him to obtain an assisted suicide?

Dialogue A

I now had what was needed to start building Eduardo's file. I then approached him and solicited all his attention. Mindful not to overwhelm him with the procedure requirements and also aware he had to be the author of his letter to Dignitas, I agreed with him we would establish a long dialogue spaced out over many days in numerous small meetings. I asked him tons of questions. I asked him the same questions many times but each time in a different manner. I invited him to remember and to qualify many moments of his present and past life. I encouraged him to speak about what he was living and to express what he was carrying inside himself. I ceaselessly interacted with him in all kinds of ways in order for him to disclose to me little by little all the elements his letter had to contain.

The first day of our sessions I asked him:

"Why do you want to die?"

"Because I am fed up with this life of shit."

"Why do you say you have a life of shit?"

"It is obvious, come on!" he answers me by indicating in a precise but jerked gesture the wheelchair in which he is seated.

"All right, but can you say it in words?"

"I can't take it anymore with the wheelchair."

"OK... Tell me, how is your life shit?"

"In everything."

"How do you spend a day?"

"I wake up in the morning and I just want to go back to sleep."

"What do you do during your days?"

"I do computer. I kill time and that is all. I cannot do anything alone. That is shit!"

"What would you like?"

"Not to be handicapped. To have a normal life like others."

"What are you missing most?"

"A girlfriend... friends."

"Why don't you have friends?"

"Because of the cardiopulmonary resuscitation."

There now we had started the preparatory work to his draft letter. Eduardo was sure of himself, unshakable. I was moved to the bottom of my soul. We had just begun the last stage of our unbelievable odyssey. I was still unaware of the many detours awaiting us on this road, but I was by Eduardo's side and I would follow him until the end.

Beside his written request, he also had to provide a sufficiently detailed autobiography to allow the doctors to assess his personal and familial situation. We had our work cut out for us...

The Capacity for Discernment

I communicated with Dignitas several times by email and once by telephone. I needed precisions. Communications have not always been fluid, but I was finally successful in obtaining a clear answer saying, "if medical reports confirm the ability to discern, we consider it is possible to prepare for an assisted suicide." I concluded with certainty and satisfaction that even if under a guardianship regime, one could benefit from the option of assisted suicide provided by Dignitas. What a relief... However, the capacity for discernment had to be established by a physician specialized in psychiatry.

I had no choice: I had to start looking for a psychiatrist who would accept to evaluate Eduardo's competence in making the decision he had made. Before anything, I wanted to know what exactly "capacity for discernment" meant in the Swiss medical jargon, what main elements were expected to be found in the psychiatrist's report confirming Eduardo's competence. And so I sent another email and, without waiting for Dignitas' response, I continued my research on the web...

In Switzerland, "a person is capable of judgement within the meaning of the law if he or she does not lack the capacity to act rationally by virtue of being under age or because of a mental disability, mental disorder, intoxication or similar circumstances" (Swiss Civil Code, art. 16). The capacity for discernment is thus presumed in every patient until proven otherwise. It is defined as the capacity to understand one's predicament and the diverse means of solving one's problem, to analyze the pros and cons of each viable option according to one's own values and to express a solid choice. The capacity for discernment is not always easy to evaluate, but it is essential for obtaining a valid consent to treatment and for the writing of advance medical directives. Therefore it is formally examined when there is a well-founded doubt concerning the patient's capacity to decide for themselves, and even more so when the decision can have important or irreversible consequences. But careful! It is not about verifying if the decision made is in accordance with the treating team's point of view or the socially conveyed values, but rather to make sure the person is able to reach a choice according to a rational decisional process. It is the patient's comprehension and competence in a particular situation at a precise time in their life that are evaluated.

Consequently, can we conclude someone is not capable of discernment only based on the fact that they have not reached the age of majority or that they are very old? No. Can we say someone is devoid of the capacity of discernment if they make an unexpected choice or a choice contrary to the doctor's opinion? No. And if someone is diagnosed with a cognitive, neurological or psychiatric ailment, is this sufficient to declare this person incapable of discernment? No. Of course not. Those are totally unacceptable prejudices falsifying the evaluation even before it begins.

How is the capacity of discernment evaluated? Not everyone agrees on the best way to proceed with this delicate examination. There are tools (tests and questionnaires) that can facilitate in some way the clinicians' task. Nevertheless, it is without any doubt in meeting with the person, during structured clinical interviews, that the capacity of discernment can be best assessed. It is a rigorous process that must be personalized and that requires time, attentive listening and empathy. In deep exchanges with the person in a dialogue friendly environment, the evaluator can properly estimate the patient's competence in the four decisional dimensions or abilities: understanding, appreciating, reasoning and communicating. Besides, the doctor doing a patient evaluation must be aware of their own limitations and keep clear of having their own judgement capacity influenced by their personal opinions or convictions or by the fear of medico-legal consequences. It is all about the patient's well-being!

Concerning the requests for assisted suicide, one can say they are part of the realities care providers are bond to face nowadays. At the time of these very particular requests—which remain, I believe, a threatening challenge for most physicians—

the applicant's capacity of judgement is, of course, thoroughly evaluated.

In Québec, we do not speak of capacity of discernment but of capacity to consent. It is the same concept expressed differently. On the Québec Public Curator website, one can read that under our Civil Code every person, including the one under a guardianship regime, is presumed to be able to consent to or to refuse care, in other words, to make a decision concerning their health. A person's inviolability and right to integrity are not cancelled by a protection measure; and even in the case of incapacity to consent, the person must always be consulted for all questions concerning them, in order to respect their autonomy. In matter concerning capacity and incapacity, it is fundamental to distinguish between the three levels of capacity, that is to say, capacity to take care of oneself, capacity to manage one's affairs and capacity to consent to health care. Regarding this issue, a decisive judgement rendered in 1996 confirms that the capacity to consent to care must not be evaluated in function of the person's predicament but rather "in function of their decision-making autonomy and of their ability to understand what is at stake."

Evaluating the capacity to consent is in fact a doctor's usual task, since this capacity is the basis for informed consent. There was a time, not so far away, when doctors made the decisions unilaterally exclusively relying on their duty of beneficence toward patients. The question of patient capacity to consent to the treatment was not even raised. But, fortunately, times have changed and, in the last few decades, informed consent has—in principle—become the central axis of the interaction between patient and doctor, acknowledging the patient's right to self-determination. According to Québec legislation, "no one may be made to undergo care of any nature, whether for examination, specimen taking, removal of tissue, treatment or any other act, except with his consent" (Québec Civil Code, art. 11). To be valid, consent must be given in an informed, free and voluntary way. To consent one has to be able to do so (it is evident!), whence the necessity for the doctor to make sure the patient manifests the four abilities necessary for decision-making. Since there are no strictly defined criteria for incapacity, doctors must rely on their clinical judgement to explore the competence of their patients. Here like elsewhere, they can also resort to guides and widely recognized work in the field. The Québec health professionals have at their disposal, among others, the Nova-Scotia criteria to verify the patient's understanding of their health problem: 1) does the patient understand the nature of their illness? 2) does the patient understand the nature and the purpose of the treatment? 3) does the patient understand the risks associated with the treatment? 4) does the patient understand the consequences of foregoing the treatment? and 5) does the patient's condition undermine their capacity to decide?

This whole doctor-led approach establishes itself naturally in the midst of the therapeutic relationship—or at least it should be so—between care provider and patient, an open relationship where an honest exchange of information must occur and where everyone must take their responsibility into their own hands. Is it possible to otherwise arrive at an informed decision contributing to the patient's well-being?

What is happening in the field in our current health system? This is another story all together.

Dialogue B

I absolutely did not doubt of Eduardo's capacity for discernment. In spite of all the neurological sequelae left by the cardiopulmonary resuscitation (CPR) that limited him in so many ways, he perceived people and situations in a stunning manner. He had already made important decisions in the past. More than once he had shown not only his capacity to contemplate a situation, to reflect and draw conclusions but also his capacity to put his decision into practice with determination and perseverance.

Well before he was 18, he had accepted surgery on his left foot. He had attentively listened to the orthopedic surgeon's explanations and had clearly understood what it would entail for him: surgery, stay in the hospital, weeks of being immobilized with his leg in a cast and afterward sustained rehabilitation exercises. But the tendons lengthening would correct his foot deformity and would allow him to stand up. Hence, he would be able to participate in his transfers and do therapeutic walks. And this for him was worthwhile. The following year, at his own initiative he asked the orthopedic surgeon to treat his left arm with Botox injections, because he wanted to increase mobility at the wrist level. He had been given a glimpse of the possibility of another surgery, but he had preferred a less risky and less aggressive approach.

At the age of 15 he had decided he would quit school. He had explained to me that he felt in prison and that there was nothing of interest for him besides music. He had considered the implications of his choice and appeared sure of himself, ready to become the organizer of his days.

It is also he who chose to do adapted karate and physical conditioning. He had one goal in mind (to walk again) and was taking the means to try with all his strength to give back to his body the agility, the coordination and the suppleness it had lost. An example of decision and of determination.

He knew what he wanted. And even if sometimes he would "spanishize" a French word or inversely "frenchicize" a Spanish word, he was able to express his thinking very clearly—at least for the interested interlocutor. I knew this ultimate decision he had just made had been deeply maturing in him. It was a cry from the heart, the expression of his whole being's burning need.

Then, one day, I resume the dialogue with Eduardo:

"Can you repeat to me the decision you have made for your life?"

"Die."

"Die?! But how are you going to do that?"

"I will ask medical aid in dying."

"And what are you going to do to get medical aid in dying?"

"Go to Switzerland."

"Very well. You are going to go to Switzerland to get medical aid in dying. What is it exactly this medical aid in dying?"

"Assisted suicide."

"Do you know how it is done?"

"They put me on a drip line with a medication."

"It's the doctor who gives you the medication?"

"No. It's me. I open the valve."

"What is the effect of the medication?"

"Rrrrr...," he answers me while throwing his head backward and closing his eyes. I understand he is imitating someone sleeping.

"I see, the medication puts you to sleep and then, what?"

"It provokes a cardiac arrest."

"Tell me, why do you want to die?"

"I can't find meaning to my life," he responds so seriously one would think he is angry.

"You, Eduardo, you had a normal life until the age of 6. What happened at that moment?"

"I had a cardiac arrest and I was resuscitated. That is why I am in a wheelchair."

"How would you describe your life after you were resuscitated?"

"A calvary," he finally says, a little aggravated (I must say it is not the first time I ask him this question).

"How do you see the future?"

"I don't have a future," he says with a sombre face.

"So you have seriously considered your situation and you've reached... I mean, what are the different options before you?"

"A or B. Go or stay."

"Tell me about option A."

"If I go to heaven, I stop suffering."

"OK. Is there any bad sides to this option?"

"No."

"And option B?"

"To stay here, it means to continue with my calvary."

"Is there any good sides to option B?"

"No."

"If we could find you a place where you would be taken care of very well?"

"It is not enough," he says firmly.

"If we were attending to all your needs?"

"It is not enough," he answers me back even more firmly, raising himself in his chair and giving me barely the time to finish my question.

"OK. What would it take for you to stay here on earth?"

"Walk."

To walk... it meant everything for Eduardo. It meant to regain all he had lost with the cardiopulmonary resuscitation.

To recover the harmonious movements of a body obeying his impulse.

To recover the ability of a dynamic brain sustaining his thinking.

To be able to move freely and go wherever he wants.

To be able to experiment, make mistakes, learn and grow.

To be able to work, create, play and love.

To be able to live in freedom and become who he is.

He could not consider continuing to exist on earth without this: to walk.

In Search of a Psychiatrist

I needed to find a psychiatrist who would accept to meet with Eduardo, to explore the course of his life, to ascertain his situation and to listen to his request, and afterward to confirm his capacity for discernment regarding the medical aid in dying he was asking for. Because, of course, there was not any doubt concerning his personal competence in the matter. Ultimately, the psychiatrist I would find would only have to devote a small portion of his or her time. And I would not ask for charity; I would pay for this professional assessment Eduardo absolutely needed.

Rejecting the idea I was maybe embarking on a perilous endeavor already doomed to failure, I went back to surfing the internet, inhabited by an immoderate hope... and I found a list of psychiatrists in private practice in Québec and also some references in Montréal.

I also contacted a cousin of mine who is retired, a trustworthy person who understood perfectly Eduardo's situation. Since she knew many people working in the field of helping relationships, she could probably put me in touch with a few resource persons.

I thought of the psychologist I had met at Eduardo's school and I looked her up on FaceBook. Maybe she knew some psychiatrists or she might have colleagues who did?

I also had the idea to locate former companions from Sherbrooke Medical School. Even if it had been ages since we had left university (would they remember me?), I would knock at their door without any embarrassment.

Many are the people to whom I talked. I had prepared myself well before approaching them, for I wanted to explain Eduardo's situation as best as possible, always keeping him, of course, anonymous. I wanted to present carefully Eduardo's perspective and transmit to them the gravity and the magnitude of the predicament he was in. I was looking for someone who would, with some humanity, extend a hand to my son.

I did not start with the first name on my list, instead with the fifth, a psychiatrist well spoken of. She listened to me sufficiently for me to explain the situation, but she rushed to tell me she was in pre-retirement and did not take in new patients. In face of my insistence, she did not soften her stand at all; on the contrary, she repeated that, even if it was not about therapy, she was really trying to reduce her work load and could not meet the person I was talking about. It was not starting very well!

The second person on my list had been retired for a few months. He advised me to contact the Psychiatry Department of the CHU (University

Hospital Center) and the Enfant-Jésus Hospital, where this kind of evaluation is done.

The third person I called was concentrating her practice in psychotherapy; what I was asking was not in the scope of her practice. She nevertheless showed understanding, and we talked at length. For a few moments, I even believed she was going to accept helping us. But at the end she refused and referred me to a colleague of hers.

This said colleague was the dry and serious type. She had been in private practice for some time and definitely did not want to get involved in a matter that risked bringing her legal problems—so she said. But what was she afraid of?

I communicated with a few other persons via email. I waited in vain for almost all the answers. But one day someone from Montréal answered me. This person "under time constraints" was offering me a consultation at her private clinic to discuss this complex subject. I immediately understood I had knocked at the wrong door.

Having arrived at the last psychiatrist on my list, and realizing the poor evaluation he had received on a satisfaction website (that I am not in the habit of consulting and that I do not really trust), I decided to drop the matter and not call him. I knew it would lead nowhere.

I then went back to my internet search with a renewed spirit, telling myself that the psychiatrist I was looking for did not need to be working in private practice. Why would there not be in the public system a psychiatrist willing to do some good works besides his usual professional activities? And I found the names of three persons.

Two of them conveyed their refusal to me through their secretaries. As for the third one, she kindly returned my call telling me that in the health system there is a procedure to follow for this sort of evaluation and that first the family physician must be consulted. This process can take months—and even more! Unquestionably, it was really not going well.

Many weeks had passed since my first conversation with my cousin when she got back to me with some good news. She was giving me, through an ex colleague's brother-in-law, the names of a few physicians specialized in psychiatry.

But the good news was not good for long. An email was left without an answer. A letter was sent back to me after several days. Someone was offended by the fact that I had allowed myself to contact her on the recommendation of a colleague she had not seen in a long time. And then, the worst: a psychiatrist apparently expert on the subject of capacity—with whom I was able, against all expectation, to speak on the phone—declaring that if someone is under a curatorship regime, we already know they do not have any capacity. With such a statement, I had good reasons to question seriously the discernment capacity of this psychiatrist, don't you think? Furthermore, I restrained myself from hanging up on her. At this stage of my investigation, the painful sensation I was looking for a needle in a haystack had undeniably taken hold of me.

Nevertheless, it was out of the question for me to give up. I therefore persisted in my prospecting task and I finally found the work place of two former fellows from the Faculty. To one, whom I had only known from a distance, I sent a short letter by registered mail to which he never replied. For the other, with whom I had rubbed shoulders at the students' residence, I had to use several means (telephone, email and registered mail) before managing to connect with her. I finally had the opportunity to speak with her on the phone. It was a long conversation. Without really knowing why, I suddenly felt comfortable with her and I told her it was about my son. I briefly related his tragic story. I do not know if she was touched by this, but she admitted to me she was not at ease with this kind of evaluation; so, she referred me to an internist who practiced medical aid in dying at a Montréal hospital. I was really fed up! Was it possible there was nobody here to come to Eduardo's help?

I then decided to contact the Québec association for the right to die with dignity (AQDMD). I told myself it would give me the chance to get in touch with several people intimately linked with the field of MAID and to set out again on a better course. Actually, it was, I was afraid, our last possibility, our last hope to find a psychiatrist who would accept collaborating with Eduardo's project. But that did not prove to be easy.

I called a first doctor, Dr Jean-François Daigle. I was very nervous before dialing the number, but as soon as I heard him at the other end of the line and started speaking, I had the pleasant sensation of conversing with an old colleague. Dr Daigle devoted lots of time to me and listened to me as I was explaining Eduardo's situation and what he had been living since his resuscitation. I told him:

"In reality, Eduardo has been agonizing since he was resuscitated, he is in an end-of-life situation since November 20, 2002, the day of his cardiac arrest. The natural course of things? For him, it was to die at 6 years of age, not to spend the rest of his days in a state of total dependence. How can we have done that to him and now refuse the deliverance he is asking for? He has the right to reclaim his death, he who has had no life for almost 16 years."

Dr Daigle understood. He understood very well, but the law as it was conceived would never allow, he told me, for Eduardo to benefit from MAID. The very small hope I was nourishing in the depth of myself had just vanished. Could he refer me to a psychiatrist who would accept to evaluate Eduardo? No, he did not know anybody, but he conversed with me openly, sharing his experience and his point of view and providing me with a lot of information.

Following Dr Daigle's advice, I contacted a law firm that could give me some more information about resources in psychiatry. The lawyer who took care of me, Mr André Payot, received my request with professionalism. He asked me to specify many things to him and he made explicit many others to me. He took care to explain clearly to me the state of affairs in Québec regarding MAID, quoting Article 15 of the Civil Code (which refers to substitute consent in case of incapacity) and emphasizing that the person I was representing always had the option to undergo a thirst and hunger strike in order to become admissible for MAID. To add this torture to all the others Eduardo had been enduring for so many years? No, thanks. Mr Payot therefore put himself to work. He was efficient and fast. But he was neither magician nor genie of a marvelous lamp, only a lawyer. The only psychiatrist he could find would accept the task we were offering him under the condition everything would be done with the support of the lawyer's office and according to a very precise methodology. That would entail revising in its entirety Eduardo's medical file (which was in Spain) and subjecting him to standardized tests. A report would be presented only if the evaluation was positive, meaning if the psychiatrist considered Eduardo was able to consent. The cost of the process would easily reach $3000 and this without counting our travel expenses between Québec and Montréal. It was heart-wrenching.

However, I was not giving up. One day, after many attempts, I found the contact details of a doctor who could certainly help me in my quest. She had given a conference on the subject of capacity and consent to care, and I was hoping that with all her experience she could direct me. In her response to my email, she was apologetic for not being able to provide me with a psychiatrist name, but she confirmed that a person under curatorship can themselves give consent to a treatment, including MAID, and she was asserting that, "a conscientious psychiatrist should make the evaluation without prejudice on the condition and the care requested." Relief? Not really, since there was no psychiatrist on the horizon.

I then contacted another doctor, Dr PierreViens. It was the second time I was calling him. I wanted to confirm a few things with him and more specifically ask him if he knew a good psychiatrist, someone understanding and open to MAID. With much frankness, he told me that often a psychiatrist's intervention in the picture only complicates things and that first you have to make sure it is absolutely necessary. I took his word for it, but it was not helping.

Searching so much and finding nothing, I was getting out of breath and starting to feel very deeply the anguish that had for months infiltrated our daily life. Most of all, I did not want to worry Eduardo with all the rejections I had met with, but I was incapable of lying to him. And a day came when I had to go over the question of the psychiatrist with him:

"You know, Eduardo, it is not easy to find a psychiatrist wanting to help you with your project. You have to pray that I find one."

"What do you think I do while taking my bath?" he answers me hastily.

"Perfect, so... but... can you imagine what will happen in one year if I do not find a psychiatrist?"

He makes gestures I understand, but I insist he verbalize his response:

"You will have to kill me and then to kill yourself," he responds with disarming serenity.

"Ah yes?! And how do you want me to kill you?"

"Easy, you buy Fentanyl on the black market."

"Well... I see you are determined to leave, but this is a very violent and dangerous option."

He agreed with me. I did not want to explore the horrible possibility he had just evoked (and which we had already talked about), and I continued the conversation:

"When you meet the psychiatrist, he will have to make sure that you are not depressed. You are not depressed, are you?"

"No, but I will become so if I do not receive medical aid in dying," he firmly answers.

"OK. There is something else... It is possible the psychiatrist thinks it is your mother who put this suicide idea in your head. What would you answer?"

"It is me who make the decision and only me!" he retorts with impressive confidence.

That was clear.

Yes, for Eduardo everything was very clear. As for me, for months I had been plunged in a seemingly impenetrable obscurity, becoming even more intense with time and oppressing me each day a little more. I was almost despondent.

And then, a glimmer of hope broke through the darkness tormenting me. At the end of a beautiful and colorful autumn day, I had the immense pleasure of having a lengthy phone conversation with the one who was to become an important ally in Eduardo's project, Dr Georges L'Espérance, president of AQDMD. From this moment forward, the anonymity in which I was keeping Eduardo vanished, for Dr L'Espérance did not want to limit himself to speak about "the person I support." Therefore my fears dissipated, and I admitted to him I was Eduardo's curator and his mother. I explained everything to him and I answered his questions. He was taking notes. I felt immediately that, this time, I had knocked at the right door. Yes, on his side he was going to search for psychiatrists and come back to me later with the results. When he told me he would also come to our home to get to know Eduardo and assess the situation by himself, I could not contain my joy! I almost cried, so intense was the emotion.

It is thanks to Dr L'Espérance that the road opened up before us. He pointed out to me that the association Exit might not have the same requirements as Dignitas and that it might be worthwhile to test the waters. I already knew, and I told him, that Exit was offering its services only to Swiss citizens, that only Dignitas was accepting persons from other countries. But I was mistaken. In going back on the web, I did find there was another organization that also was welcoming foreigners: Growing Path.

Growing Path was founded in Basel about ten years ago. It is committed to the respect for human dignity, the right to self-determination and the legalization of assisted voluntary death in every country. Among Growing Path's priorities are maintaining and improving quality of life, as well as suicide prevention, although its main objective remains patient self-determination, especially at the end of life. The admissibility criteria for assisted suicide and the costs are the same as Dignitas.

In less than a week there was quite a turnaround. I called back Dr L'Epérance to give him the news: he did not have to look for a psychiatrist any longer. I had contacted Growing Path by email and the president, Dr Gisela Kosch, had confirmed to me it was not necessary for the capacity of discernment to be evaluated by a psychiatrist. Wonderful, was it not? Now, we needed him to confirm Eduardo's capacity of discernment.

I repeated to him that Eduardo was determined. I also wanted him to know what Eduardo had recently asserted, “There is nothing in my life that is worth my staying in this world.” He had made up his mind in late February 2018 and his decision remained firm over time. Dr L’Espérance graciously accepted the delicate task I had just given him, and we fixed a date for the first meeting.

I felt immensely comforted. On our solitary road, we had found a friend. This was heartwarming.

Dialogue C

I was so relieved... After months spent on an empty search for an understanding and empathic psychiatrist, at last I was seeing an opening, the real possibility for my son to progress on the road that would lead him to the realization of his project. When I informed Eduardo of my headway, he quickly understood a huge obstacle had been eliminated. He did not say much, but the expression I saw on his face said it all. He was very satisfied. We both felt reassured by the turn of events, and suddenly the air we were breathing became lighter. I took this opportunity to come back to our talks and I asked him:

"Can you tell me about your suffering?"

He remained silent for a long while. I realized I had not asked the right question. So, I started again:

"On a scale of 1 to 10, where 1 means no suffering at all and 10 means a lot of suffering, where would you place yourself?"

"Nine."

"Nine? That means you suffer a lot."

"Yes."

"Why 9 and not 10?"

"Because there are times when I laugh."

It was true. I still heard him laugh out loud almost every day, when he watched cartoons or comic shows.

"But why do you suffer?"

"I am suffering physically, intellectually and emotionally," he affirms somber and serious altogether.

"Physically, why?"

"Because I am sitting in a wheelchair all the time. My body doesn't obey me. And I have a lot of myoclonus."

"And intellectually?"

"I can't read, study, work..."

"And why do you suffer emotionally?"

"I don't have a girlfriend and I don't have any friends."

"I understand very well that you are suffering enormously, Eduardo. It hurts me to see you suffer, you know. What is the best thing that could happen to you?"

"Another cardiac arrest."

And this time without resuscitation, please!

"So, you don't have hope for the future?"

"Do you see any light in my eyes?" he retorts, his face tensed.

No, I did not see any.

This short tête-à-tête dictated by the circumstances had allowed Eduardo to verbalize his ache of living. I was struck by the way he was able to express his suffering. I knew well how difficult it was for him to articulate words and to put sentences together with some fluidity. In spite of my efforts to remain serene before him, I was feeling at my core in a very special way the wound we both had been carrying for so many years. But, at the same time, I was happy to hear him speak once more with the lucidity that was his, and I was hoping he would show the same eloquence in his encounters with the physicians.

Preparing the Dossier

From the moment I contacted Dr Kosch, everything went very fast.

Even before receiving Eduardo's complete dossier, she grasped the magnitude of the situation in all its dimensions and extended her hand to us. She understood the great suffering preventing him from living. She asked me to send her a short film so that she could see Eduardo a first time. Sure! I also received from her solace I had not expected and that soothed me a lot, "What good mother you are, it is so difficult for a mother to accept and to respect this wish from her son!" She told me this after answering all of my questions with clarity and precision. I was touched. I already knew without the shadow of a doubt that with her we were heading in the right direction. I was happy to be able to continue working with all my strength for the choice Eduardo had freely made.

I told Dr Kosch that Eduardo would have liked his suicide to be on November 20, the same date as his cardiac arrest in 2002, but that it was not possible because of Air Transat flights availability. I also told her there were two things he wanted to see happening before leaving: the publishing of our book *¿Por qué me han reanimado?* in French and in English and one last trip to Spain to again see his friend Paz. He had therefore decided his assisted voluntary death (AVD) would be in August or September 2019.

First of all, Eduardo had to become member of the association. On November 6, 2018, he signed, in a rudimentary way (EDU) but with a firm hand, the Growing Path membership and living will forms, which I had filled with and for him. Two days later, I informed Dr Kosch we were seriously thinking of September 5, 2019 for Eduardo's AVD. The next day, after giving me some additional information, she answered me that she had made a "provisional reservation for 5.9.2019 for Eduardo." It was wonderful! Eduardo's project was beginning to take shape...

Nevertheless, we had to make an official request for AVD according to Growing Path's requirements. We needed Eduardo's medical reports summarizing his diverse stays in hospital in Spain. Where had I put them? I looked everywhere in our apartment; I searched and searched again many, many times, until I decided to open an envelope labeled "Copies of everything I sent June 5, 2013." Bingo! At that time, some judiciary proceedings were taking place in Córdoba between me and the father of my children. I had sent my lawyer all the original documents likely to be useful in her pleading before the Family Court judge. Among the copies I had just discovered were those of

Eduardo's medical reports. Without delay: email to my former lawyer, search for the originals in my thick file (contentious divorce) and mailing of these precious documents. A certified translator from Montréal made the official translation that had to accompany the originals. I told myself that after translating Eduardo's medical reports, she might want to know the sequel of his moving story. So I took the opportunity to suggest she read our book. After reading the excerpt available on Amazon, she sent me an email, "Your story is simply astounding. Eduardo's journey, even read through the medical file, is heart-wrenching." We were happy she had bought the book. We had touched another person.

The dossier also had to contain a recent medical report. We needed to be prudent for we wanted to maintain Eduardo's project in the strictest confidentiality. I told our family doctor we were thinking of going back to live in Europe—which was not totally untrue, for I had already thought of it many times in the relatively recent past—and I had to assemble a complete dossier for my handicapped son. The other difficulty was that our family doctor did not know Eduardo very well, since he was almost never sick and that, as he took pleasure in saying, he was benefiting from the care of his personal doctor, that is to say me. To fill in this gap, I provided her with all the information necessary to write a detailed summary of Eduardo's medical history. We were truly very fortunate to be able to count on the collaboration of our physician. Eduardo was not giving that much significance—certainly because he trusted me 100% in managing the whole process—but I was greatly pleased about that. The Swiss physicians who would read the report would have a very good idea of Eduardo's global situation even before meeting him.

The time had come to proceed with the evaluation of Eduardo's capacity for discernment. I wanted that to happen as soon as possible, because you never know what could complicate things when you least expect it. As nobody is sheltered from an accident or a stroke... Fortunately, everything took place without a hitch. As he said, Dr L'Espérance was able to easily arrange to come to our place, in Québec, in the midst of his frequent traveling between Montréal and Bas-Saint-Laurent. Assisted by his partner, also a physician but retired, he evaluated Eduardo in two steps: in two lengthy formal meetings, he assessed Eduardo's state and his life circumstances in depth, as well as the non-ambiguous perception he had of his own existence.

Dr L'Espérance went straight to the point. Immediately after the greetings, he more or less addressed Eduardo in these terms, "Your mother told me you have decided to go to Switzerland for an assisted suicide. Can you tell me why?" The answer came without delay, "Because my soul is suffering." But Dr L'Espérance did not understand at all, for Eduardo had a great speech and utterance impediment. One needed to be used to his way of speaking to understand him. So Eduardo repeated, "Because I am suffering" and I also repeated after him to make sure the message had been well received. I think Dr L'Espérance was not expecting such an answer. As for me, I was looking at my son and I was seeing him equal to himself: succinct and substantial.

Dr L'Espérance noticed right away the spastic quadriparesis limiting all of Eduardo's body. And then, as he explored, he observed that he totally lacked equilibrium, that he did not control well any of his movements, that he had abnormal reflexes, that each of his gestures was frustrated by all kinds of neurological alterations (dystonia, dysmetria, athetosis and myoclonus) and that he could not carry out any daily or domestic life activity. In short, he was completely dependent on others. Yes, he noticed the terrible sequelae constraining Eduardo's body to permanent and final disability.

Dr L'Espérance observed as well Eduardo's capacity to reflect and to express his thoughts. He realized that in spite of the brain damage, Eduardo perfectly understood his situation and his neurological state. Eduardo told Dr L'Espérance he was suffering because he was in a wheelchair without being able to do anything by himself. He told him he did not want to continue living like this and that he wanted to die to end his suffering. And he spontaneously added he was mad at the doctors for what they had done (resuscitating him), because he could be in heaven. He then told him about our book, which told his story and would soon be published in French.

For Dr L'Espérance, there was not any doubt about Eduardo's capacity of discernment, and this was apparent from the first moments he spent with him. In his remarkable report, encompassing the notions of informed consent and of capacity to consent relating to MAID in Québec and Canada, he concluded that despite being under guardianship, Eduardo had the absolute right to his self-determination. He also mentioned many observations proving Eduardo's capacity to ask the right questions and to make an informed and thoughtful decision about his future. I read Dr L'Espérance's report with heartfelt and profound emotion. This document was of invaluable importance for Eduardo's project. I was happy for my son.

At the end of November 2018, Eduardo's request for AVD was received by Peaceful Bridge, the foundation associated with Growing Path dealing with requests made by members for assisted voluntary death. Of course, there was no absolute guaranty. "I can never give you 100% assurance he will be accepted. He must have the medical visit in Switzerland, before we can only be 99% sure," answered Dr Kosch, whom I was now calling by her first name, Gisela, as if she was a friend – which she had already become! In order to complete Eduardo's dossier, we needed to send, six months prior to the AVD, scanned copies of some legal documents required by the Swiss authorities: birth certificate, passport, proof of residency, sworn statement of celibacy and the report confirming the capacity of discernment.

I prepared our trip to Switzerland in two shakes of a lamb's tail, at lightning speed! We had to make reservations while there was still room on the airplanes and in the hotels! For our last flight together, I bought tickets in Club class. We enjoyed a lot consulting the menu offered by chef Daniel Vézina on Air Transat. Confident, Eduardo chose an entrée of duck comfit lasagna. Judging by the expression illuminating his face, it was as if he was already relishing the dish. Since I did not know the hotel where we would be staying, I called before making reservations for our room to make sure there was wheelchair accessibility. I also wanted to be certain I would be able to maneuver easily with Eduardo in the bathroom. With the plan provided by the hotel, I could check that there was enough space and that the combination bath-sink-toilet would not hamper our movements. The trip was booked, what a satisfaction! Eduardo's project was moving forward without a glitch...

But something kept bothering me: the capacity of discernment. Was Dr L'Espérance's report sufficient? In consulting with Gisela again, I realized the opinion of a second doctor would contribute greatly to the solidity of Eduardo's dossier. Without delay I turned to Dr Viens and I called him a third time. He would really have been sorry, he told me, if I had asked him to support Eduardo's request for MAID here in Québec. Indeed, he would have been forced to refuse, for it would have been absurd to participate in an endeavor with no chance of succeeding. But since it was about collaborating with a well matured project that would be taking place in Switzerland, Dr Viens offered his help with no hesitation whatsoever.

Eduardo might not be at the end of life for society, he remarked, but I have the impression he sees himself as such and this is all that matters. He was probably right. I then shared with him what Eduardo was often saying, that his life had ended when he was six and that his hell had started with the resuscitation. I even repeated to him word for word what Eduardo had told me again a few days earlier, "I am a living fossil, I died but I was forced to stay."

Before Dr Viens came to our home, I checked with Eduardo an option he had talked to me about, complete voluntary fasting. I had my own opinion on the subject, but I wanted Eduardo to freely express his view. I repeated to him what Dr Viens had explained to me: that a way to become admissible for MAID was to stop eating and drinking (this is considered as refusing treatment) until one is in an end-of-life situation. In front of such a possibility, Eduardo said only one word: horrible. This was clearly not a tenable scenario. Luckily!

Dr Viens admirably grasped Eduardo's situation and produced a report that marvellously supported and completed Dr L'Espérance's. Reading our book, which he told me he had devoured, was paramount for him to understand his journey and his state of mind. He said that Eduardo was cognitively very present, and he noticed the active interest he was manifesting in his surroundings. He observed that in spite of the communicating problems (dysarthria), he could build an argument, debate it and defend—sometimes vigorously—his ideas. He also sensed in Eduardo the frustration and the anger fostered by the impossibility of foreseeing significant social relationships, even the smallest ones. His dearest dream, to walk, was inaccessible and his other dream, to have a girlfriend, would never come true. His condition was irreversible and he knew it. He told Dr Viens, talking about assisted suicide, that "this will take me to Heaven."And then, in a theatrical manner, he mimed the process of his assisted voluntary death.

When Dr Viens asked Eduardo if he understood the risks associated with assisted suicide, Eduardo started laughing quietly and answered, "I am not afraid." He also told him about the possibility of a positive outcome in the proceedings concerning the laws on MAID, which could render him admissible here, in Canada, and save us from a costly trip to Switzerland. Eduardo let him know in no uncertain terms that he did not want to wait, that it had to happen in 2019.

Dr Viens saw very well that Eduardo was aware of what was happening around him and the life full of meaning and of interesting things the other youths of his age were enjoying. He saw he could reflect by himself and that he had made a final decision based on his own reality. Eduardo knew that without assisted suicide, he would continue to suffer like he had for the past sixteen years. And that was out of the question for Eduardo.

Conclusion: two experienced doctors were declaring that Eduardo had full capacity to decide regarding his request for assisted suicide. I could not ask for more. All of my search efforts had borne fruit at last. Eduardo's liberation process was progressing little by little... And as strange as this may seem, I was looking forward to the ever more approaching death of my son. Was it not the deliverance he was wishing for?

All that remained for me to do was submitting the legal documents to Peaceful Bridge at the opportune time and making the payment for the AVD approximately two weeks prior to our departure for Switzerland. I thanked Heaven hundreds of times for getting married in community of property.

Thanks to the sale of the house we had lived in in Spain, which I owned at 50%, I could myself finance Eduardo's project.

Dialogue D

It was often during or after supper that we engaged in our true conversations, that we took time relating to one another. One evening, he told me point blank:

"Life is worth living and it is better not to have to take your own life. But there are situations when this is what needs to be done."

"What kind of situations?"

"Situations like mine."

I understood him so much... But I said nothing. I remained silent. He then declared on a sharp tone:

"Me, I walk again or I am out of here. Since it is not possible to take back my former life, I choose to leave."

Clearer than this, impossible. I wanted to emphasize to him that his assisted suicide would have consequences on the people around him. His answer came out like an arrow:

"Why don't they all go to hell! It's me who decide, my life belongs to me!"

"But you realize you are leaving me alone, abandoning me in this world?"

"Yes."

"And it does not bother you?"

"No," he responds with conviction, "I have already told you, only one person could make me stay."

Yes, I knew. For Paz he would stay here, but under the condition, of course, of being able to walk.

We continued talking about his liberation process. He then brought up on his own the notification of his passing to his father, insisting that I must do it only when everything would be finished. He wanted to be sure nobody would interfere with his project. I reassured him saying:

"Don't worry, Eduardo, when the time comes I will explain your point of view to him."

"My departure has already been spoiled once, it is not going to be spoiled another time," he added with much emotion in his voice.

Dear Eduardo, he would have liked so much to live his life... During the last months before his passing, he expressed many times, always with the same vehemence that characterized him, that the life he was living was not his, that his life—his own true life—had ended when he was six years old, that he had been robbed of his life and of his death also.

The Letter to Peaceful Bridge

During each of our conversations, I faithfully recorded all that Eduardo was telling. I jotted down numerous drafts that I corrected multiple times according to the author's commentaries. After a while Eduardo came to write, always with my help, his official request to Peaceful Bridge. Here is the content:

"I am Eduardo García Beaudoin. I want to have medical aid in dying. I am asking Peaceful Bridge to help me to go away with an assisted voluntary death.

I am fed up with the life I have. I would like to have been born a long time ago, when cardiopulmonary resuscitation did not exist. In this way I would not have been resuscitated when I had my cardiac arrest on November 20, 2002. I could be in heaven and I would not have to live this calvary every day. I go to bed at night and I would like to never wake up again.

I do not have a disease. I am handicapped because of the resuscitation. I am in a wheelchair. My body does not listen to me. I lack balance. I do not control well my movements and I have a lot of myoclonus.

I cannot do anything by myself. It is my mother who dresses and undresses me; it is my mother who brushes my teeth and shaves me; it is my mother who helps me at the toilet and it is even her who wipes my bottom; it is my mother who washes me; it is my mother who helps me to eat; it is also her who helps me to do my transfers; it is my mother who accompanies me for my fitness sessions; it is my mother who handles the television remote control for me; and it is my mother who reads to me, etc. Life with my mother sucks; but it is better than to be in a nursing home. I do not want to go rot in one of these places.

I cannot take it anymore with this life of shit. I wake up in the morning and I would like to keep sleeping. I kill time with the computer. Sometimes I play games; sometimes I watch cartoons or comic sketches; sometimes I listen to music. I have physical conditioning 2-3 times a week with my mother's help. In the evening I watch television with my mother. It happens that I go out for a ride with my motorized wheelchair with my mother, but it is rather frustrating because it really does not ride very fast.

My life is not a life; it is a calvary. What I would like is to walk. I would like to do everything by myself and as I feel like doing it. I would like to stop being handicapped. I would like to have a girlfriend, go out with friends, play football, go biking, go on forest hikes, read and write, learn things, work, play piano, go rock climbing, drive a car. I would like to be free. I would like to pee like a man, eat by myself, lie down on a couch and channel-surf as I wish, fool around my way, go where I want to when I want to. I would like to be with my girlfriend to protect her and to do all I can for her. I would like to live a real life. But it is not possible. It will never be possible. I will never be able to do any of all those things.

I had a mission: it was to try to walk again and take back the life I had before. I did all I could for that, but it did not work. I am still in a wheelchair. I have no autonomy. I have no freedom. I have no independence. And I am fed up to live like that. Staying here, it means to continue living in hell, it means to continue suffering... suffering physically, suffering intellectually and suffering emotionally. The best that could happen to me is another cardiac arrest.

I want to die because I cannot take it anymore with the wheelchair. I want to die because my life has no meaning. I want to die because I cannot do anything. I cannot be who I am. The future for me is to continue with the same calvary I have been enduring for years (16 years). I have had enough. I do not know what it means to live with dignity, but I would like to die with dignity.

If I leave with an assisted voluntary death, I am going to heaven. It means I am freeing myself from my handicap, it means I stop suffering. This is what I want. I need Peaceful Bridge to help me die."

The Autobiographical Notice

We took time to reflect on life as it had flowed. We travelled in the past and the present; we visited many heart-wrenching moments; and then, the most important events that had marked Eduardo's life and which he wanted to tell were naturally laid down on paper. Here is the autobiographical notice Eduardo presented to Peaceful Bridge:

"My name is Eduardo García Beaudoin. I am 22 years old. I was born on August 6, 1996, in Córdoba, Spain. My father is a Spaniard and my mother is a Quebecer. I was an energetic and dynamic boy. I had started to do judo and I loved playing football. During the summer I spent hours in the pool. I liked going to school and I had my group of friends. There was a girl in my class I liked a lot: Paz. I still love her.

On November 20, 2002, I had a cardiac arrest at school. I was resuscitated and taken to the hospital. After two weeks, I came out of the Intensive Care Unit in a vegetative state. It was over. I had lost everything. I was screwed. It is my mother who helped me to get out of there. With her I worked for years. I went through all sorts of treatments: physiotherapy, speech therapy, multi-sensorial stimulation, osteopathy, equitherapy, hydrotherapy, percutaneous fibrotomies, Botox treatment, surgery, adapted tricycle, therapeutic walks with adapted walker, etc. I recovered some things, but I am still in a shitty situation: I am in a wheelchair, my body does not listen to me, I have no freedom, I have no autonomy.

My parents divorced three years after my cardiac arrest. My mother wanted to stay in Spain, but my father would not let us live in peace. So we left for Canada. It was August 2008. My older brother chose to stay in Spain, but he also came to Canada two years later.

At the beginning we were living with my grand-mother. When she sold her house, my mom and I, we moved into an apartment. My brother went to live with his dog in another apartment. I only see him a few times a year. Anyway he does not care about me. My father sends me a book on my birthday, but I do not have any contact with him since 2015.

I do not have friends. Nobody communicates with me. I have my mother. And I have an aunt who accepts me and understands me. Her name is Martine and she lives with her brother Jean, who has Down's syndrome. I go to their place, in the country, twice a month. It is there that my dog Luna lives because dogs are not allowed in our apartment. I miss her every day.

Here, in Québec, I spent five years in a specialized school, but I did not like it. Nothing interested me. Everything was decided and controlled by others. I had the impression of being "in prison." I was glad to be able to quit school when I got to be 16. Since then, it is me who organize my days. I do computer: music, games, cartoons, documentaries, humoristic sketches, video-clips and FaceBook. I often listen to music. It helps me when I feel I am going to explode. I pass time. All I do is this: passing time.

I have been training for seven years 2-3 times a week at the PEPS (sports pavilion) of Laval University. I was hoping to walk again one day. That is why I have done physical conditioning for years. I truly believed that putting a lot of efforts long enough, I would succeed in changing my situation. Today I know that nothing will change. I am before an insuperable wall. If I continue to train it is to keep my strength.

In 2015, I asked my mother to write my story. It's important that everyone get to know what has happened to me. I do not understand why I was resuscitated. My life is not a life, it is a calvary. I hope that my story will open the eyes of many people and mostly the doctors'. The book, my mother wrote it in Spanish; and soon it will be available in French and English on Amazon. I hope many people will read it and will start reflecting on resuscitation. I really hope to be heard.

But anyway this will not change what I am living. For me there is no hope. I will continue to suffer in my body and in my soul. I will continue to endure the same calvary every day. I will continue to be alone. I will continue to be imprisoned in my damn wheelchair, without being able to do anything by myself. It makes no sense for me to continue like this. It makes no sense to stay in a world where I can't live in dignity and in freedom. If I do not walk, life has no meaning.

With my mother I will do a last trip to Spain in May 2019. I want to see again my native country and Paz. After that I will be ready to go.

Besides my mother, there are two other persons who know what I am going to do: my aunt Martine (the one with whom my dog Luna lives) and a cousin of my mother. The two of them understand that I am suffering a lot and that I want to be over with. As for my brother, I will tell him at the last minute.

I will travel to Basel with my mother and maybe also with my aunt Martine, but it is not sure she will be able to come.

Life is worth living and it is better not to have to take your own life. But there are situations when this is what needs to be done. For me what I am living is unbearable; and so I am happy to be able to go to heaven."

The Last Times

We came back from Spain on May 21, 2019, at the beginning of the evening, tired but gratified. We had just spent two weeks in Córdoba, Eduardo's native town, and we were deeply delighted with this unforgettable journey. The climate had pampered us with its spring sun caressing our skin without burning it and the lovable freshness of its evenings, and every day we had not missed any opportunity to indulge ourselves, savouring the delicious dishes of the Spanish gastronomy. The two of us, without being gluttons, loved to eat—it is still the case—and each of our culinary adventures had made us happy. But this was not the most important. What made our stay really extraordinary was that Eduardo could make his desire to see Paz again a reality. He even saw her more than once.

Paz, his beloved. She was more precious than the apple of his eyes. She was his jewel, his priceless pearl, his fabulous treasure. He was keeping her tenderly in his heart. She inhabited tenderly all of his thoughts...

Eduardo had bought a gift for his friend: a double chain that could be worn as a necklace or as a bracelet, very pretty, of elegant simplicity, formed by two ranks, one of fine gold links and one of minute turquoise stones. A delicate jewel that would sit beautifully on the one who was reigning in his heart. To accompany his gift, he had asked me to make a special card using one of his colorful mandalas, a task I had executed swiftly with an overwhelming enthusiasm, thanks to an image manipulation software installed on our computer. Inspired by the love songs he was listening to every day, he had composed very tender words for Paz, words emerging from the depth of his being, from his innermost recesses, from his soul, from all he was, words living and vibrating in him.

During one of their reunions, Paz asked Eduardo how he was spending his days since he had arrived in Córdoba. He answered with his deep voice, intensely looking at her, that the most beautiful thing of his stay was her. She melted. Together they shared a cocktail, a soft drink, an ice cream, another cocktail, and another... Every meeting was an immense joy for Eduardo. And for me. I cannot describe in words the sight so sweet and so beautiful I had the privilege to witness each time they met. Eduardo devoted himself to contemplate Paz. He would plunge without shame his caressing gaze in the one he loved. He would invade her with his piercing eyes again and again. He would literally drink her with his gaze. I will never forget it.

When Gisela told me she was going to Vancouver at the end of May 2019 to participate to a conference on MAID, I mentioned to my sister Martine, jokingly, that she could as well at the same time make a stop in Québec. "What are you saying?" she exclaimed. Of course, I was not really counting on it; it was asking too much from Providence, but nothing prevented me from imagining this soothing scenario. Some time later, to my great surprise, Gisela sent me an email announcing her coming to Québec, for she wanted to know Eduardo before our trip to Switzerland. What satisfaction! What comfort! She was coming here, to our home, to meet Eduardo, to ascertain his situation and to make sure by herself he was capable of discernment. On learning the news, Martine, hiding her worry regarding the outcome of this visit, exclaimed, "Wow!" I was jubilant.

The meeting was planned for Saturday afternoon May 25, as soon as they would arrive in Québec. Gisela was accompanied by Lukas, her life companion. We gathered together in our living room with an invigorating coffee and a slice of cake I had backed specially for them. Without losing time, Gisela plugged in her laptop computer and went to work. She was seated with Lukas on one of the small couches, and Eduardo, whom I had just introduced to her, was in front of her, sitting in his wheel chair, waiting, docile, for the interrogating to begin.

Gisela energetically opened the conversation. She had a goal in mind: to corroborate, as a Swiss physician, the conclusions arrived at by the two Canadian doctors. From the start of the exchange, she asked me not to intervene too fast—which I was doing, without being aware of it, to remedy the communication difficulties. What was happening was between her and him, and I understood she wanted to preserve her interaction with Eduardo from any interference that could falsify the evaluation. Evidently. In my feverish state, I had not realized how eagerly I was shouldering Eduardo. So I adjusted myself to the circumstances, withdrawing gently to the background, but remaining attentive, ready to repeat or translate Eduardo's words.

As she was exchanging with Eduardo, Gisela was taking note of everything she was gathering. I remember observing with astonishment the agility of her fingers dancing on the keyboard and the impressive speed at which the file opened on her computer screen was filling up with her home visit report. Finally, she lifted her head up to Eduardo and, satisfied with her observations, confirmed that he could go to Switzerland for an assisted voluntary death. Eduardo was not surprised; he was sure of himself. On my part the relief was huge; I was starting to breathe truly better. We had just passed a crucial step in his liberation process.

The evening of the same day, we celebrated our rejoicing and raised our glasses with Gisela and Lukas, whom I had invited to partake of our humble supper. And the next day, we all gathered together in our apartment around Eduardo: Dr Viens, Dr L'Espérance and his partner, Gisela and Lukas and myself, of course. To cheer up our meeting, I had prepared things to nibble on, but nobody touched anything. Everybody was too occupied in discussing MAID. As for me, I did not resist a few chips and a glass of white wine and, moved, overwhelmed and grateful at the same time, I enjoyed watching this singular scene: my 22-year-old son, destroyed by medical technology, surrounded by four doctors who were supporting him in his endeavor to obtain an assisted suicide. On the very difficult road of Eduardo's project, I felt pampered.

After Gisela and Lukas' visit, there were only three months left before Eduardo's AVD. A last summer together. We lived it as we were used to live, one day at a time. We did not seek overdone entertainment or try to do extraordinary things, like exorbitant outings, capricious purchases or gastronomic meals in the best restaurants of the city (except for the flight Montréal-Basel in Club class, which was not extravagant at all viewing the exceptional circumstances). We truly continued to live each day very simply, faithful to ourselves, in fully enjoying the delicious moments—too few in number—of our dismantled life. Eduardo did not even ask me to prepare him a special drink, already tasted or to be discovered, he who was nonetheless a lover of cocktails.

It was not particularly hot that summer, but we still spent many weekends at Martine's and Jean's, in Cap-Saint-Ignace, refreshing ourselves in our rustic swimming pool. Eduardo also needed to be with Luna, his cherished dog, to feel her very close to him, to look at her and to caress her, to cling to her in his jerky but very tender hugs. Luna, without knowing anything about Eduardo's project, seemed to understand what was happening and would abandon herself to his insisting embraces with a remarkable docility.

When we spent the weekend in Québec, I would do something special for the Saturday evening meal; I would give our cook (me) her day off and, already relishing myself for Eduardo, I would go to get some chicken at St-Hubert rotisserie. He would always choose the same thing: a chicken leg roasted with classic Portuguese spicy seasoning and piri-piri sauce, preceded by cheese sticks with a Marinara sauce dip. He loved that and I was happy, every time, to see him lick his fingers.

Eduardo continued to train at the PEPS with the same assiduity. He never missed a day in the rhythm naturally established throughout the years. One week, he would go Tuesday, Thursday and Saturday; and the following week, he would drop Saturday for we would go to Cap-Saint-Ignace. And so forth until the last day. Very often, it was during one of his bodybuilding sessions or while riding in the car that he would share with me his reflections. One day, at the end of an exercise, he told me, "From the decision I have made, we can say I have all my mind." Exactly. A little later, on another machine, he added, as if it were a sentence, "I was robbed of my death!" I could only concur. And shortly before our departure for Switzerland, this time in the midst of his efforts to lift a weight, he rightfully declared, "If life is sacred, let's stop interfering with it. Death is also part of life."

On July 8, 2019, we had our last outing in the woods. The prospect of a ride with Eduardo in his motorized wheelchair has always been for me a source of great stress. This time was no exception to the rule. I installed Eduardo on his vehicle, I took my courage in both hands and we went out. I knew that for Eduardo, this stroll—like all the excursions we had made in the past—was the occasion to drive his engine dominating the space in his very peculiar, somewhat disorderly way. For once, it was for the others to adapt, not for him! I understood him. While being super vigilant, I kept the promise I had made to myself of not reminding him of the security instructions. His experiencing a little freedom was much more important to me than a perfectly performed circuit.

In the past several months, Eduardo had ceased coloring mandalas on paper and would not leave the computer. Except when I needed it. I would then take his place in front of the screen and, while I would manage diverse affairs, he would use his iPad to do puzzles and virtual coloring. On the computer, he would continue to play games and to listen to cartoons, preferably in Spanish, but it was mainly music that engrossed him. Varied melodies filled with emotions tirelessly invaded our apartment day after day, taking him to another universe and allowing him to escape somehow from the unbearable heaviness of his existence. So when we noticed a billboard advertising the movie *Menteur* (*Liar*), with Louis-José Houde, we decided to go to see it, just to break the monotony. Eduardo thought he would laugh a lot, but that was not the case. Disappointed, he only gave this production a rating of 5 out of 10. I was saddened that this evening had not given Eduardo what I would have love so much witnessing. But thanks to *Menteur*, we saw that another interesting movie was showing: *Hobbs &*

Shaw, presented by Fast and Furious, starring Dwayne Johnson, Jason Statham and Idris Elba, three actors he knew very well. On August 19, 2019, we went back to the Odeon Cineplex in Ste-Foy for what was to be a memorable performance. The movie is an action-packed, original and breathtaking composition, an explosive mixture of unending fights, exciting pursuits and verbal confrontations seasoned with caustic humor, so uplifting that Eduardo almost fell off his seat more than once. He was thrilled, and I was happy to see him enjoying himself, especially when he gave me his verdict: 10 out of 10. A great success he would have asked me to buy on DVD.

I made good use of the small camera Martine gave me as a birthday present some years ago. It seemed to me appropriate to keep audiovisual documents of our conversations, and I told Eduardo I could film him while he was answering my questions concerning his life and his project. He was on board. We made a lot of videos, most of the time improvising, and sometimes in a more structured way. Even if these films are creations of an unskilled amateur—and so of poor quality—the recorded moments remain of great value to me. Quickly, I took a liking to the camera and I decided to capture Eduardo at different times of his daily life. Therefore I have some moving souvenirs of him that are very dear to me. I can now see him again eating, trying to move forward in the pool, playing with Luna or caressing her at night before going to bed, transferring with me from his bed to his wheelchair or vice versa. And as well, I unwittingly recorded bits of his humor, a vivacious and contagious humor that still makes me laugh today.

I remember one evening, at the end of the month of February. I was opening the mail of the day while Eduardo was eating. I had received an off-sized envelope whose sender I did not recognize. I was intrigued. Discovering what it was about, I commented out loud, "Ah! These are the slips for your income tax return!" Instantly, Eduardo replied, "Did I become more expensive?" We laughed.

During the last two weeks before our trip, I reviewed with Eduardo all the stages we had gone through working on his project and went over the important aspects of what was awaiting him in Basel. Often but gently he showed himself to be exasperated by my questions. Nevertheless, he understood he had to seriously prepare himself to face the last verifications that would take place before his AVD. At the end of our repetitions, I asked him:

"Are you sad to go?"

"Why would I be sad?" he retorted as if my question was superfluous.

"Ah... I understand. When I announce your departure, people will ask me 'Why did he do that?' and me, what am I to answer them?"

Suddenly, Eduardo became all tensed and with emphasis declared something I did not understand at first. He willingly repeated:

"I don't give a damn what they might think. It is my life, it concerns nobody but me. They leave me alone!"

He was right. He did not have to justify himself in the eyes of others.

A few days before flying, I talked with him about a hypothetical situation. "Imagine that God appears to me and that I could..." I started to tell him without being able to finish my sentence, because he immediately interrupted me:

"God tells you He can grant you two wishes!" he said energetically.

"Ah yes? What wishes?"

"To give me back my legs."

"Yes, of course, Eduardo. And what is the other wish?"

"That He give me back all of my intelligence."

"Dear Eduardo, if only it were possible, I would give up my entire life, I would completely disappear, for you to regain your life."

Eduardo was very conscious of his limitations. He was suffering immensely in all the dimensions of his being. Is it not horrible to be imprisoned in one's own body? Is it not horrible not to be able to live but only to survive? Is it not horrible to be left at the mercy of others?

Yes, his soul had been horribly mutilated. Constrained to an empty and meaningless existence, each instant was for him an unbearable suffering.

Fortunately, we had worked very hard for years and, in spite of his handicap, Eduardo had grown into an adult able to exercise his right to self-determination, to assert himself, to take a decision for his life and to make it become reality. A truly great victory... a real miracle!

A Transcendent Love

Is there anybody on Earth who could live without love? Is there anybody who could deprive themselves of any relationship and be happy? Without love, is life worth living?

Eduardo loved Paz with all his heart and with all his soul.

But his mutilated body had become a prison preventing him from conquering her in this world, to take her with him to protect her from any danger and to cherish her forever.

He kept his love pure and burning in the depth of himself. Chained in a monstrous solitude, ripped in the very essence of his being, he did not know what it means to love and to be loved on Earth.

He was not able to free this flame burning him from within, this boiling spark filling his heart, but he succeeded in touching his beloved in another dimension.

I heard him sing to her his love and, in listening to him, I perceived the intensity of his feelings, the fervor of his passion, the intoxicating echo of the throbbing of his whole being turned toward her.

"Where are you, my sweetheart, where are you? I need your love to live!"

"As a ray of light penetrating the darkness, you entered into my life... I am so imbued with you that I feel a fire inside me, a fire burning me, a fire inflaming me, a fire slowly devouring my heart..."

"Today I looked for you and I found you in my dreams... I am a thief, for I would like to steal you, my beautiful flower... this kiss might be for me my reason to live..."

"Tell me only that I am your most precious gift... and without a doubt, I will give you my whole life..."

"I think of you, I spend my time thinking of you... Teach me how to listen to your lips, how to read the sun; take me where dreams fabricate your voice. I think of you, I rock my soul thinking of you..."

"It is so painful to live, it is always painful to live without you; I need your scent, I need your warmth... I love you forever, my love."

"Without you, it is better not to live... without you, why exist?"

"You are going away, you are going away, leaving me without saying anything, without offering anything. Let me weep for you in a corner; it will be better this way, I know it. I have forgotten what you were for me; now I only feel an unending pain..."

"I want to sleep in your eyes and, on waking up, drink from your mouth; for of you I am still thirsty... I will be your air; you will be the skin covering my solitude... I want to be by your side!"

"You will always be in me, even if I never see you again; my heart is weeping for you... in the sky, there is a star resembling you, shining like you... You will always be in me!"

"I look at you and the impossible becomes possible; I look at you and I am intoxicated by the magic of your presence..."

"My tears are today these verses your absence will never erase... You have left in each corner of my soul small pieces of your heart... Goodbye, my beloved, I am going away, I am letting you leave, I will never forget you..."

He said the best that had happened to him during his stay on Earth was Paz.

And in her heart, beyond the world separating them, she has, I believe, welcomed his love simply, in sincerity and in complicity with him, in this other dimension.

Eduardo loved Paz with all his heart and with all his soul.

His love was boundless. I feel it still vibrating...

The Last Days

Before leaving for Switzerland, Eduardo and I had agreed that we would, as soon as we arrived, modify the rhythm of our life so as to gently move toward the day of his AVD. Used to going to bed at the wee hours of the morning and to get up when everybody is already in full activity, we had to adjust again to a schedule concurring with that of the people around us. Fortunately, the fatigue from the trip would facilitate the necessary change for us.

The day of our departure, it seemed as if someone was trying to put a spoke in our wheels. I had reserved an adapted taxi to take us to Pierre-Elliott-Trudeau Airport. It all started when the taxi driver chose to use the highway 20, where we met more than one hindrance, one of them with sufficient magnitude to raise in me some concern. Then, we found ourselves in incredibly dense and slow traffic on the outskirts of Montréal, where a lot of road work was being done, which delayed us enormously and further worried me. To top it off, the driver did not even know the route to the airport! He took the wrong way! We had to make a detour and stop at a gas station to ask for directions. I thought we would never get to the airport! Finally, we arrived on time for registration without trouble, but... as we were quietly waiting at the boarding gate, an annoying voice coming out of the speakerphone announced the flight was being delayed. We patiently waited two more hours before boarding the plane!

Once settled in our seats, I told myself that nothing else could stop us from taking off. I was not mistaken. Eduardo was comfortably seated with his seat belt buckled, and I could relax at last. Happy to fly toward this destination with no return for him, we avidly started enjoying the perks of our flight in Club class: a small glass of wine, orange juice, appetizers... We were already flying!

After savoring his duck comfit lasagna and his dessert (layered white cake garnished with raspberries, if I remember correctly), Eduardo was ready to watch the movie he had selected: *Aquaman*. He had already seen it, but he really had lots of fun reliving the moments of action, of fanciful adventures, of humor and of love this last movie was offering him. When the plane landed at the Basel-Mulhouse-Fribourg international airport (EuroAirport), still full of energy, he screamed victory, "Did you see that? I did not sleep all night!" He was glad and proud.

We arrived at the Spalentor hotel later than planned, at the beginning of the afternoon, on August 31, 2019. A very nice young woman led us to our room. Horror! The bathroom was so exiguous that we could not enter it without touching the walls. With much kindness, the hotel employee went back to the reception desk computer to check the room availability. In visiting a few empty rooms and finding it was impossible for me to maneuver with Eduardo in any bathroom, I felt, helpless, anxiety regaining power over me. Shit! Was it possible that Eduardo be deprived of his bath during his last days in this world? Thank Goodness, in inspecting the third room, I recognized the bathroom whose plan had been sent to me by email months earlier. "That is the one, yes, yes, it is the bathroom I saw, this is our bedroom!" I exclaimed, smiling, relieved, very grateful for all the efforts the young woman had made to satisfy us.

We quickly took possession of our little temporary nest and we went out to meet Basel, this charming Swiss town where Eduardo would be able to pass away in peace.

Equipped with a small map of the town and a public transportation pass we were given at the hotel, we went to the stop to take the tramway in direction of the old city, just beside the Spalentor, a monumental gate from the Middle Ages, vestige of Basel's ancient walls. I did what the young woman at the reception desk had explained to me: in seeing the tramway approaching, I started gesticulating to attract the driver's attention onto Eduardo, a new user in a wheelchair. The driver stopped the tramway, got out and installed the access ramp. As I was carefully loading us into the car intended for us, I indicated to him the station where we would get off, "Barfüsserplatz," in English "Franciscans Square," a central location where several tramway and bus lines intersect. Eduardo laughed at me in hearing my voice awkwardly pronounce this German word. I laughed with him.

It was nice outside. It was hot. The sun was shining in the sky. The streets were swarming with people attending to their occupations, be it work or leisure. The town was greeting us, was smiling upon us, was welcoming us. Lighthearted, we started on the way that would lead us to Mittlere Brücke bridge, which we were thinking of crossing to go for a stroll along the Rhine. Suddenly, I noticed Eduardo was no longer holding himself in his chair; he was nodding off! No wonder with the trip we had just made. Thus our walk had just fallen through and we needed to go back to the hotel to rest. But we were not going to bed on an empty stomach. In no time, we took a seat at an outside table on a restaurant terrace, improvised on the stone pavement, and we cheerfully shared a plate of fish and chips, accompanied by an orange soda for Eduardo and a beer for me. It was delicious!

Back at the hotel, we perfected our technique for the bath in this new environment that was now temporarily ours. I thanked Heaven for still having the strength and the agility to become one with my son and to help him slide into a foreign bathtub... and get out of it! I was truly happy that Eduardo could soak to his heart's desire in soothing, relaxing, calming warm water.

That night, we slept like satisfied and comforted children, falling into a deep and regenerating sleep.

The next morning, fresh and renewed, we left the hotel to undertake—this time for real—the last of our earthly peregrination. Like the day before, we exited the tramway at Barfüsserplatz. From there, we strolled slowly in the already busy streets following the simplest way to the Rhine. My sense of direction being what it is (which is non-existent), I did not want to take any risk. Such a feeling of freedom took hold of me as we were crossing the famous Mittlere Brücke bridge. From either side the sight was superb; a light breeze full of sun was tickling our faces; and I was moving forward wheeling Eduardo, a smile on my lips, dauntless, fully aware of the place where we were. Each hour, each minute, each second that passed was taking us closer to Eduardo's liberation. I was throbbing.

Every day we went wandering on the marvelous promenade laid out along the Rhine. We familiarized ourselves with the Rhine in one way and in the other, each time discovering a different landscape. That Sunday, the first day of our tourist excursion, we met an old lady walking her dog. She was sitting on a bench, alone, and was watching the little curly ball sniffing around. On seeing us, she smiled vivaciously and spoke to us a few kind but incomprehensible words. Responding to this nice invitation, we stopped to keep her company a few minutes and, despite the language barrier, we chatted with her a good while. We explained to her that we came from Canada, but we were also Spaniards, that we were visiting for a few days, and we also told her about our dear Luna. She seemed to understand. Eduardo was glad to hold the small friendly beast on his knees and to give her treats the lady was gently putting in his hand. The dog was wiggling with pleasure under the tender eyes of her mistress, visibly very moved by this moment of closeness we were living together. Of course, a little further, I could not help taking a wet wipe and erasing the dog's caresses off Eduardo's hands. As we were pursuing our route, we remembered our walks along the Guadalquivir, in Córdoba... but what a difference: here, in Basel, there was water in the river!

The streets were rich in restaurants, taverns and bistros of all kinds, and any tourist was spoilt by choices. But not us. We needed to find a place where the washroom was wheelchair-accessible. And so we were restricted in our gastronomic experience. However, we managed very well and discovered the ideal spot to savor our dinners: the hotel Merian restaurant, located at one end of the Mittlere Brücke bridge. Their menu of the day, composed of an appetizer and an entrée (without dessert), was very affordable—taking into account the exorbitant price for anything in Switzerland—and their outside terrace overlooking the Rhine offered us an enchanting setting. We were well served in every way.

Our first complete day in Basel ended in one of the only restaurants in the vicinity of the hotel that opened their doors on Sundays. We shared a veal fricassee served with rösti, a typically Swiss potato galette. Eduardo wanted to water down his meal with a *calimocho*, a drink Swiss people do not know. So I ordered a cup of red wine, a Coca-Cola and a glass with ice cubes to prepare this Spain-flavored beverage for him. Delicious supper.

Upon returning, I noticed Eduardo had a stuffed nose. Firmly denying he had a cold, he told me not to worry. He seemed sure of himself, but, knowing him by heart, I relied more on my observation. That night, I fell asleep unable to overcome the fear he would get sick just before his AVD.

The cell phone rang. With the strange impression of having slept very little, I got out of bed, confused. It was still dark outside. I told myself that at 6 a.m. with a cloudy sky, it was normal. I took my shower; I woke up Eduardo, who showed his usual collaboration; then we got dressed and went to the cafeteria, which was on the fifth floor. But to our great surprise, the door was closed and locked. Weird. I looked attentively at my watch: it indicated 1:07. I thought however it was about 7 o'clock! Suddenly, I understood. Having been unable to switch my cell phone to local time when we arrived, I had left it at Québec time and I had programmed the alarm accordingly, that is to say at midnight to get up at 6 a.m., Basel time. What happened is that in the mean time the phone adjusted itself automatically to local time, without my noticing it! And the alarm rang at midnight, Basel time. The only thing to do was to go back to bed. Eduardo could have got mad at me for taking him out of bed in the middle of the night, but I was lucky: he did not fuss at all, restraining himself to kindly laugh at me and at my unfortunate mistake.

On waking up, I no longer had any doubt: Eduardo had a cold. In normal time, I would not have done anything for he preferred ignoring the cold and getting better with no special intervention on my part. But this time, facing the impressive schedule of the coming days, I thought it was better to convince him to let me treat him. Before undertaking our wanderings for the day, I bought in a pharmacy a bottle of sea water I would use to irrigate his upper respiratory tract several times a day, which might give me a chance to defeat the naughty virus.

We could not skip over the visit to the Botanical Garden, located just in front of the hotel where we were staying. We went around it with interest; I took the time to read to Eduardo many of the cards accompanying the different specimens—some very exotic—inhabiting the garden. We made a pleasant pause, Eduardo always in his wheelchair and me on a bench, to simply let the sun penetrate us with its comforting rays, to enjoy the calm and the perfumes emanating from the plants around us. What particularly captivated us, I must say, is the encounter with two intriguing characters from the animal world: a very elegant small lizard wisely camouflaging itself in its rocky environment and a minuscule frog with flamboyant colors that, on spotting us, in a few quick leaps disappeared in its pond garnished with beautiful water lilies. On this vibrating note we ended our visit.

We went back sauntering along the Rhine and, that day, we saw something rather unusual: there were human heads attached to floating orange balls being carried away by the current. "Look at that, Eduardo, people are swimming in the Rhine!" I immediately thought of my sister Martine, who does exactly the same thing but in the river Bras Saint-Nicolas, in Cap-Saint-Ignace. Except that she does not have at her disposal any *wicklefisch*. It is a waterproof and resistant bag, fish-shaped, conceived specially for swimming, a good example of Swiss ingenuity. Baseliens use them to stow and keep their clothes, towels and personal belongings dry while taking it easy in the refreshing waters of their magnificent river. The orange balls were *wicklefisch*. If it had been possible, I would have bought two of them and I would have thrown myself with Eduardo into the adventure... The inconvenience was that we could not put the wheelchair in a *wicklefisch*!

Our meeting with Gisela was scheduled for 6 p.m. that day. Punctual, we had come back much earlier and were patiently waiting, Eduardo concentrated on his iPad and I sitting in an armchair, when the phone rang: Gisela was telling me she would arrive shortly and that Dr Josef Hausmann, her psychiatrist friend—whom she had asked to accompany her during the interview—was already installed in the hotel garden. We immediately joined him to greet him. He was a man of the third age, calm, relaxed and jovial, someone simple inspiring confidence; he did not speak French very well, but he understood it. We had only exchanged a few sentences when Gisela joined us; and, without further delay, we all took refuge in our hotel room, sheltered from prying eyes and ears.

Needless to say how happy we were to see her again. She was coming with the same dynamism I had perceived in May, vibrant, light, resolute, but she had a skin rash partially covering her face, neck and arms. The difficult law suit she had been subjected to was the cause. In his fight against assisted suicide, the canton attorney had accused her in 2016 of homicide and non-respect of the law on therapeutic products. Even if she had finally been acquitted of the homicide accusation in July 2019, she was to appeal the other charge. Three years of legal proceedings and it was not over yet! I was deeply sorry, saddened by the fact she was attacked in this fashion. In spite of the threat weighing on her, Gisela had accepted to help Eduardo. It was a gesture of such generosity... Eduardo told her, "You have a big heart and you need a good lawyer to protect you."

In one corner of the room the four of us formed a tête-à-tête, Eduardo in his wheelchair, Gisela on the edge of one of the beds, her psychiatrist friend in the armchair and I on the desk chair. Gisela had to make sure Eduardo had not changed his mind, that he was certain of his decision and that he was acting freely. She also wanted her psychiatrist friend to witness Eduardo's competence. So, once more, some questions... Eduardo answered without hesitation, with his habitual vivacity, with serenity. Dr Hausmann was impressed by his performance. In spite of all the limitations his handicap was imposing on him, Eduardo was able to get his message across; the amazingly strong expression we could see on his face and the gestures, not very fluid but full of sense, he was joining to his poorly articulated discourse did not leave any doubt in his interlocutors' mind.

During the interview, Gisela's phone vibrated. She took note of the message with a worried look. Her friend asked her if there was a problem and, nodding, she responded she needed to call Lukas back as soon as possible. Interested, Eduardo asked her a question, "What color is your problem?" She answered tit for tat, "It is of black color!" And I was marvelling, once more, at Eduardo's genius.

That evening, we stayed at the hotel for supper. I was feeling tired, exhausted, after Gisela and Dr Hausmann's visit; and Eduardo was really indisposed by the cold. His nose was running like a maple tree in spring time! We thus satisfied ourselves without complaining with what the hotel snack-bar was offering: a ham and cheese Panini for Eduardo and a tomato-cheese baguette for me. It was good enough.

"I have a sore throat." These words, said just before going to bed, alarmed me. Was he going to be sick precisely at this moment of his life? He did not have any fever for the time being, but... And if it worsened? How come I had not thought of buying an analgesic? Luckily, the pain was not intense, for we did not feel at all like going out in search of an on-call drugstore. Besides, it was late. So I sprayed sea water in Eduardo's nostrils; I massaged him, seeking with my energy-freeing hands to soothe him the best I could; and I prayed for the night to be as peaceful as possible.

I was answered. Thank Goodness. But, of course, Eduardo was not miraculously cured during his sleep. Immediately after breakfast, we went to the closest pharmacy to obtain some ibuprofen. We had just enough time for the medication to start acting and for Eduardo to feel better before Dr Gunther, the psychiatrist coming to see him to confirm his capacity of discernment, would arrive. This was the last professional evaluation before his AVD.

And what an evaluation! It was not just a formality to complete Eduardo's dossier, far from it; it was a serious and rigorously structured interview that had no semblance with the relaxed meeting I had imagined. When I saw Dr Gunther unfold a huge geographical map of the world, I realized the magnitude of the confrontation that would take place between the psychiatrist and my son. My nerves were being put to the test but not Eduardo's. Keeping a calm as impeccable as disconcerting, he showed his examiner he knew perfectly where he was and where he was going. Dr Gunther tested him in all manners. After ascertaining his cognitive functions of attention, orientation and memory, he systematically sounded his capacities for comprehending, analyzing, reasoning and judging. He also evaluated Eduardo's mood with a detailed questionnaire to make sure he was not depressed. I started to relax only when the interview became more like a natural conversation. At that moment, Eduardo told Dr Gunther his life was like a calvary. And he asked him, "Do you know what is a calvary?," at which Dr Gunther responded, "Of course, it is the mountain where Jesus carried his cross." Satisfied with his answer, Eduardo did not insist; he knew he had understood what he meant. The ambience had pleasantly lightened. Eduardo was getting off with flying colors and I felt serene. Dr Gunther pursued his exploration in questioning him on his decision. He then turned toward me and made the point that my life was going to change completely from one day to the next. I was happy, I answered him, with tears filling my eyes, that he had been able to choose the denouement of his tragic story. Eduardo simply added, “She will learn to live without me.” Dr Gunther, who had already put away all his materiel, took the trouble of taking out notebook and pen from his briefcase to record this reflection of Eduardo, a reflection he judged full of maturity. It was the cherry on the cake! Thus ended this historic meeting in the morning of Tuesday, September 3, 2019. Then, Dr Gunther stood up and, leaving our room, he said to Eduardo, “You passed the exam. Bon Voyage!”

We had the day ahead of us, and this time we would be roaming Basel streets permeated with a pleasant sensation of satisfaction. Our happy steps took us to Münsterberg street which leads to Basel Cathedral, whose original presence we had already appreciated when strolling along the Rhine and which we wanted now to contemplate up-close. However, Münsterberg street, being built on a vertical plane, was for us an insurmountable obstacle. I did not even dare attempting the ascent, so steep was the slope. We were wisely turning around when a couple of tourists, a Spanish woman and an Argentinian man, realizing our problematic situation, offered to escort us to the top. It was very nice of them. I rapidly considered the man: he was well built, able without a doubt to maneuver the wheelchair. I told him that if he pushed Eduardo on the way up, he would also have to push him—or rather to hold him back—on the way down. It was okay. We then started climbing together while chatting in Spanish. Delighted by this unexpected company, we went around the cathedral and even could admire a section of its interior. However, we did not enter its main part for, at that moment, there was some kind of ceremony taking place (probably a mass!) that tourists were not allowed to disturb, but the echo of the melodious canticles filling the church reached us through the ancient walls. As an emblematic figure of Basel, the Cathedral majestically dominates the Rhine and, from the terrace decorating its rear facade, we enjoyed the fantastic view it offers to all who come to visit it.

Once we had come down, we left our anonymous companions, thanking them warmly. And then, enjoying our freedom, we continued nonchalantly roaming around in the streets that already were no longer unkown to us. After dinner at the Merian restaurant—of which we had become usual clients—we went back to the hotel, Eduardo to busy himself with games and music available to him on the iPad and me to rest a little. As dessert, we devoured a few Swiss chocolates. Rich. Smooth. Refined. Exquisite. Sublime. What could be better for a sweet tooth? After swallowing a truffle, Eduardo exclaimed, "Holy shit! It's so good!"

To beautifully end the day, we decided to go back in town at the end of the afternoon to savor a cocktail. We chose a place outside where we could sip our beverage while enjoying the good weather. Eduardo told me that the cocktails I prepared for him at home were better than the one that had just been served to him. What a compliment! Thrilled, I pointed out to him that mine always contained a unique ingredient giving them an unequaled flavor: his mother's deft touch full of tenderness! He smiled. Finally, we toasted reliving in thoughts the success of the interview with Dr Gunther...

That evening we had supper in a good restaurant close to the hotel. Eduardo feasted on a plate of home-made pasta, linguine with salmon sauce, that, before my envious look, he let me taste. However, faithful to himself, he made a face when I offered him a bite of my succulent salad. I was only teasing him a little, of course. Eduardo was not picky, but he hated raw vegetable salads. And this was not going to change now, less than 48 hours before his departure.

The following day, Wednesday September 4, 2019, was the last day we were going to spend together. We left some time after breakfast, as usual, to go to the old town: getting off the tramway at Barfüsserplatz—which, after five days in Basel, I managed to pronounce with a certain ease—and new wandering improvised in the midst of a world swarming with activities, a world Eduardo was about to quit. We returned strolling placidly along the Rhine like the previous days, fully aware it was the last day.

We interrupted our walk for a long moment. In silence. We were facing the river whose waters were overflowing with life, Eduardo always nailed to his wheelchair and I sitting on a bench. Both of us pensive. He was looking afar. I was gently peering at him. I tried to say goodbye to him. I looked for the words that could faithfully bear what I was feeling... in vain. We had already said everything to each other.

The road had been long... Painful. Terribly distressing and harrowing. Hopeless. Unsustainable. All this time of connivance between us had brought us here, in Basel, on the edge of the Infinite, where his being who could no longer stand it was to fly off toward his destiny.

We needed to go back at the hotel for three o'clock in the afternoon because Natasha, Gisela's assistant, who wanted to meet Eduardo before the big day, was coming to visit us. She was an affectionate and sensitive person, with a glowing smile and a manifest talent for communication. Upon entering the room, she took a copy of our book out of her bag. What a beautiful surprise! She had already read a few passages, thus getting her close to Eduardo in a special way. We talked a lot. About his life, about his struggle. About the absurdity of CPR. And then about his AVD, which was to take place the following day. She explained to us in detail how things were going to happen. And we had her listen to an excerpt of the song with which Eduardo wanted to go into the hereafter: *Abre las puertas del Cielo*—in English "Open the doors of Heaven"—a prayer-song he had found himself in one of his innumerable cruises on the internet and that he often played at home, that he even sang with all the fieriness inhabiting him. "Are you sure?" she asked Eduardo. And he answered, "What a question!"

Gisela sent us a WhatsApp, "I have received the reports today, everything will be fine tomorrow!" It was reassuring. We could continue to quietly advance in this ultimate day.

At the end of the afternoon, toward 5 p.m., we connected with my sister Martine on FaceTime. She told Eduardo how much she admired his courage and his determination, and she thanked him for his integrity, for having lived in truth. I do not exactly recall the words she pronounced, but it's as if I could hear her tell him that it was a privilege to have known him and to have witnessed his tenacious struggle to find anew the way to his life. With a voice full of emotion, she declared to him he was her hero. Both of them looked at each other, deeply moved to the bottom of their soul. I was there, beside Eduardo, taking care to hold the iPad at the proper height, and I felt shivers down my spine. No tears were shed, but the world shook around us.

We were going to get ready for the evening when Eduardo abruptly turned toward me and said:

"I want to do some FaceTime with Paz."

"But it is impossible, Eduardo."

"I want to see Paz," he responds, determined, firm as a rock, with his face suddenly transformed by the emotions culminating in him at this moment.

He started to sob his heart out, waves of uncontrollable tremors sweeping through his body. I looked at him, distraught, torn apart by the pain of the absence that was disfiguring him, and I tried to reason with him:

"Eduardo, you know very well we can't call her. We already talked about it; it would be too risky, you know it as well as I do. Besides, she would worry to see you in such a state. Come on! Let's get ready for supper, OK?"

He kept quivering throughout his entire being, devastated by a torrent of tears. I felt like weeping with him.

"Eduardo, you can't do that to me now. I understand you feel like seeing her and talking with her, but it's impossible. You have to take hold of yourself, otherwise I too will collapse."

Nothing would do. Eduardo was weeping and weeping. What could I do? For a moment I thought I would really succumb to this unforeseen trial, but I succeeded, I do not know how, in recomposing myself and I told him:

"Listen, I know it's difficult, but you must be strong, Eduardo, I beg you. Remember the short video we prepared for her and in which you say your goodbye to her... You know what? We'll send her a WhatsApp message, if you want?"

Then, seeing there was a possibility to get in touch with her, he calmed down and nodded. I took my cell phone and I wrote for him:

"Hello, dear Paz, I hope you are well. I am thinking of you a lot. I take you in my arms and I hold you very tight."

He wanted to add at the end of the message a few emojis, one of merriment, two of love and a last one of sadness.

Once the message was sent, a certain tranquility allowed us to change our clothes and to go to the restaurant, but I could clearly perceive the fire consuming Eduardo from within and I was fearful of a new eruption at anytime.

We went to Latini, an Italian restaurant we had spotted earlier in the day, located only a few steps from Barfüsserplatz. After checking the wheelchair access to the toilet and taking a look at the menu offered, which had made our mouth water, we had decided that it was at this place we would savor our last supper. Upon arrival, we chose a table close to a window, away from the main brouhaha, where we would enjoy the intimacy we needed. I had started to read to him the description of all the very appetizing pasta dishes there were on the menu when Eduardo interrupted me all of a sudden, "I want meat." Evidently! I turned the page at once and got to the more substantial dishes. Eduardo did not hesitate; he opted for the veal cutlets with lemony sauce, served with pan-fried potatoes.

I had prepared for him a *calimocho* and the waitress had just put the most inviting plate before him. Only mine was missing for our feast to begin... And then, what could be seen coming happened: Eduardo burst into tears again. I looked at my phone to check for messages. Nothing at all. Then I undertook the task of consoling him, but it was not easy. Sincerely, I was hurting as much as he was and, moreover, I was aware that words would not do much. Without my being able to explain it, he at last quieted down and we managed, in spite of everything, to recreate a comfortable ambiance, relaxed enough to allow us to fully enjoy our ultimate supper.

Back at the hotel: the last bath. He abandoned himself in it like any other night. Calm had returned for good. Eduardo had regained the serenity he had shown all along his project. I was reassured. All was well. Furthermore, he had completely recovered from the cold. That was like him: no virus (almost) resisted him.

At the end of this grueling day, finally comforted, we slid into the last night...

The End

It was Thursday, September 5, 2019. It was the last day. In fact there were only a few hours left in Eduardo's life. I did not detect any nervousness in him. I saw him especially serious, impressive, majestic on this day when he would find again the way to paradise. He suggested skipping breakfast so we would save time and not be late. Out of the question. We had more than enough time, I remarked to him, and, besides, I absolutely needed to restore my strength. So, we ate together one last time, in silence, savoring our buttered toasts spread with apricot jam. A little delight.

It is a collaborator of the funeral parlor enterprise who came to pick us up at the hotel. The car arrived a little before the appointed time, but we were already all set, waiting beside the little garden in front of the hotel. Eduardo was wearing the clothes he had chosen: his jeans and his white tee shirt, a gift from his aunt Martine, adorned with a beautiful picture of Paz and him. He was going to leave this world with her on his chest. Fresh shaved, with his goatee carefully brushed, perfumed with a fragrance from Calvin Klein, the nails clean and well cut, his hair au naturel, he was handsome.

The taxi was driving a white SUV; its floor was thus higher than the one of a standard car. In spite of this, I succeeded without too much difficulty in installing Eduardo on the passenger seat. I disassembled the wheelchair, which we put in pieces at the very back, and I sat on the rear seat with my packsack.

Direction: Lausterberg, at about 30 kilometers south-east of Basel.

The sky was covered with a layer of light grey clouds that nonetheless let us guess the coming sun break. After what seemed to be a long time, seeing we were penetrating more and more into unknown territory, Eduardo asked while looking at the driver, "Does he know where we are going this guy?" Of course, I answered him. Not only should he know the route, but he also had a GPS. So...

Nevertheless, having arrived at the destination, we felt we were lost. We were at the end of I do not know where, in what resembled a small clustering of old businesses dissimulated at the heart of a somewhat quasi clandestine zone. The driver, who spoke German and thus could not tell me anything, stopped the car. I could see he did not know where to go from there, that he had no idea of the way to take to lead Eduardo to the place of his final departure.

We got out of the car, he and I, and we scanned the surroundings. Nothing. With signs I made him understand to call Gisela's assistant—who had herself assured me of her entire availability for any problem that could arise—but only the answering machine answered. I then asked the driver, this time with impatient gestures, to call Gisela, who had to have her cell phone activated. The driver dialed the number I had just indicated to him from my contacts list. Awaiting an answer, he was listening, paying attention, waiting for someone to pick up at the other end of the line, looking at me with an inquiring face... but not saying a word! Nobody was answering his call! The two phones were on voice mail!

Then I started to panic. Really. Anguish took hold of me and, for an infinitely long moment, I thought everything had fallen apart.

Eduardo, who was still in the car, did not perceive, I believe, the state of alert in which I was. He was looking at me, calm, apparently wondering what was the matter, nothing more. While the driver went to ask for information at one of the neighboring shops, I checked the address on the wall of the building the car was parked by, as well as the diverse signs posted there. We were at the right place, but nobody seemed to be waiting for us. Strange. And troubling. More than troubling, it was terrifying.

I almost lost my cool. I felt I was fainting. As if everything was collapsing. I was looking at Eduardo through the window of the car and I just did not know what to think. What were we going to do? We were alone in the middle of nowhere!

Then, suddenly, as I was turning around, I saw Gisela and Natasha who were climbing down the stairs leading to the Peaceful Bridge premises. This sight sufficed to chase away the assault of my painful worry. A big smile of relief settled on my face, and I motioned Eduardo, showing him my thumb up, that everything was fine.

Gisela explained to the taxi driver how to go to the back door of the building, where there was a ramp by which Eduardo could access Peaceful Bridge refuge. The car barely made it, so narrow was the dirt lane around the building. I put the wheelchair back together; I installed Eduardo on it; I paid the taxi and we went upstairs. Once inside, we discovered a welcoming space, consisting of large open rooms, simply decorated, where warm colors in the shade of orange dominated. Gisela's psychiatrist friend, Dr Hausmann, had come; he would be the witness to the event. They all noticed, very moved, the tee shirt Eduardo was wearing.

We installed ourselves in the back room, around a big conference table, where we held the most important summit meeting. Before anything, we had to hand Gisela the originals of the legal documents and complete the paperwork. Since Eduardo needed to sign four official declarations, Gisela took care to read them slowly to him and to explain some passages as necessary. He was filmed while signing the last paper to prove that the signature "E D U," laboriously traced in separate letters, was truly his.

Nothing was missing from the dossier. Everything was in order. We moved to the next step: that is to install Eduardo on the bed awaiting him. For the last time, I helped him get out of his wheelchair and make his transfer. I took off his shoes and his orthosis; I put the sock I had brought on his left foot; and he lay down in the most comfortable way possible.

Gisela carefully examined Eduardo's arms, one after the other, looking for a venous access. She succeeded at the first try in inserting the catheter in one of the veins of his left forearm. Once the drip line was well connected and firmly fixed (so as to prevent any shifting), the time had come for Eduardo to practice opening the perfusion valve. The people at Peaceful Bridge came up with a small device for tetraplegic persons: to open the perfusion, one only needs to press on a lever.

However, Gisela did not want to use it with Eduardo. Because of his involuntary and badly coordinated movements, someone could say that his gesture was not really voluntary. For that reason, she absolutely wanted Eduardo to open the perfusion by himself, which he was to do without anyone's help. He sat on the bed, as suggested by Gisela, and started to struggle with the perfusion. After a while, his efforts being fruitless, he threw a "Coño!," a Spanish bad word to which only Gisela's assistant (who understood the language a little) reacted. I laughed. And suddenly, he succeeded! Bravo! Gisela told him he had to try again another time. Obedient, Eduardo went back at it. It was no easy matter! Nevertheless, he had to succeed. As for me, I was a bundle of nerves. This time, seeing he could not do it, he shamelessly yelled "Tabarnak!," a bad word from Québec, to which nobody reacted, of course. I laughed. And finally, after multiple attempts, Eduardo got to open the perfusion! Wonderful! But, would he be able to do it at the moment of truth?

The tension is high. I am so nervous that I do not realize it. Calm and reassuring, Gisela takes me aside and reminds me that Eduardo needs me. She is right. Thanks to her, I can calm down. Eduardo lies down again on the adjustable bed, in semi-reclined position. I take the iPad and play the song, to which we listen with him for several minutes. We are all gathered around him, strongly united by the melody he has chosen. At his signal, I put the music on pause. He is ready. Gisela is going to ask him four questions...

... From where I stand, behind Gisela and her assistant (who is filming), I am unable to see his hands and to observe the progress of his efforts; but, suddenly, I perceive his satisfied countenance looking upward, toward the small transparent bag containing the lethal medication that starts flowing in him and that is going to give him back his death. And I understand he has succeeded in opening the perfusion. Deliverance! At last! He is free. He is soaring in Eternity...

The assistant stops filming. I turn the music back on. Gisela seizes the iPad and I concentrate on Eduardo.

I took his face in my hands and I laid on his forehead a kiss filled with all my love. Our gazes met; then he dozed off and closed his eyes...

I put my hand on his chest and I sensed his heartbeats fading away. He was going...

I took back the iPad; I stayed close to Eduardo, in communion with him; and I watched him leave... and I let the song play to the end. Gisela discretely put a candle beside him. Sobs surged from my being and accompanied the music until the last note, sobs revealing my sadness, my relief, my wonderment, the loss of my son, his sufferings and his deliverance, my joy in front of the fulfillment of an incredibly long and painful path.

With my happy hands, with my eyes flooded with tears, with my heart delivered from its oppression, with my body trembling with emotion, I went over Eduardo's carnal envelope and I tenderly replaced his feet and right arm that were immobilized in a somewhat grotesque stance. He was now resting in peace.

When I turned around, I fell in the warm embrace of the people who were accompanying us. Taking me into her arms, Gisela told me, "You are the best mother I have ever known." I thanked her from the bottom of my heart, for she had given us, to Eduardo and me, the most beautiful gift.

And then came the police and the medical examiner. I feared a little this unavoidable meeting with the authorities, but all went well; actually, everything happened with the utmost respect. The police officers were very understanding and, while the medical examiner proceeded to the ascertainment of the death with his trainees, they spoke at length with Gisela. Without comprehending what they were saying, I saw they approved of the mission she has given herself, her commitment for the right to self-determination and the help in suicide she brings to the persons who need it.

Thereafter, it was the turn for the employees of the mortuary to arrive at the premises. Three very respectful men were coming to take Eduardo's body and carry it to the cemetery. They showed much sensitivity. After offering me their condolences, they left me alone in the room where Eduardo's body was resting. Those are precious moments engraved in me forever, but it is difficult for me to describe them.

In the space of a moment, it is his whole life that unravelled... By what right was his six-year-old fragile little body assaulted when he died suddenly on November 20, 2002? How could his death be so daringly profaned? What justification could be given to the martyrdom he had lived?

After years of persistent struggle, Eduardo had at last found rest. He was lying there on the bed. His calvary was over. I was dazzled by the greatness of what had just happened. Happy for him, I contemplated him in silence. And in me resounded "Victory!"

Behind closed doors, the people from the mortuary did their work. During this time, I stayed in the company of Gisela and Natasha, who explained to me what would happen next. Gisela advised me to go to the cemetery with the mortuary employee in charge of transporting Eduardo's body. She did not think it was good for me to be alone too soon in my hotel room. In checking the location of the cemetery on a virtual map, I could orient myself adequately. The road to travel back to town was very simple and would only take one to one and a quarter hour by foot, depending on the speed of my steps. It was perfect.

Before the coffin was closed, I was offered another moment of intimacy with Eduardo. I was grateful. I looked at him intensely, filling my eyes and my soul with his image. His arms had been brought on his stomach and between his crossed hands a red flower had been placed. He was handsome. I admired him one last time with his love tee shirt... My son Eduardo was dead. Alleluia!

The cemetery was impressive: an immense and very beautiful garden sheltered by large, protective trees. A place conducive to meditation. The minivan stopped near the building where Eduardo's body would spend the next three days. Like a shadow, I followed the mortuary employee in each of his gestures. After taking out the casket from the vehicle, he put it on a stand with casters and rolled it inside. I watched him identify the coffin whose top he had just fixed. I went in with him in the cold room to the exact place where he left the bier containing Eduardo. Afterward, on a big board hanging on one of the walls of the corridor nearby, he wrote "Eduardo Garcia" in the column for September 9, 2019, the date fixed for the cremation. Then, he walked me back to the exit and left me with a discreet smile and a firm handshake.

I crossed the cemetery very slowly, invaded by a sense of ineffable plenitude. The sun had come out of the clouds that were dissipating; the weather was beginning to be nice. I went back downtown following the Rhine, moving along in the new lightness of my being, with Eduardo not anymore in his wheelchair but in me. I told him, "Dear Eduardo, we've succeeded!"

Paz answered four days later, the Sunday before my return to Canada. That day was grey and gloomy. It even rained part of the afternoon. But Paz's message came in, somehow lightening my day. She explained to us that she was traveling with her family in the North of Spain. If she had not responded on Wednesday, I thought, it was certainly because her phone was off or in airplane mode. She asked how we were doing; she said she was thinking of us; she seemed cheerful. I was happy to read her message. I answered her that we were on a trip as well and that upon return we would tell her about it... You see, Eduardo?, she has answered and she sends you a kiss!

On Monday, September 9, 2019, Mr Arnold Meyer, the funeral home director, came to pick me up at the hotel around 9:15 a.m. Even before leaving for Switzerland, I had shared with Gisela my desire to be present for the cremation, and she had made the necessary arrangements.

At the entrance of the building where the crematorium was, we waited, the director and I, for Eduardo's coffin to be brought in. The man in charge of the cremation, who spoke English, asked me if I wanted to see the deceased one last time. I answered yes, of course. Then they placed the coffin just in front of the crematory oven, took off the lid and moved away to respect this intimate and sacred moment.

I was before my son's dead body. I bent over him and, profoundly moved, I touched him. He was hard and cold. The petals of the flower he had in his hands had sagged but were still attached to the stem. I could follow on Eduardo's arms the course of the blood vessels whose purple color contrasted with the paleness of his skin. His head had slightly tilted to the right; his cheeks had hollowed. The almost solemn expression that had settled on his face transpierced me. His entire body had solidified, but it was him, Eduardo. I could not hold my tears that suddenly gushed forth; I sang to him a love song in Spanish—a melody I had heard so often, especially during the last weeks—and I prayed.

My prayers finished, I then signaled the mortuary employees and they came to prepare the coffin. I withdrew to a certain distance, as the one in charge had indicated to me, and I stood close to the wall facing the crematory oven. In only one click, the oven door opened, the coffin was engulfed and, even before the door closed, powerful flames grabbed it. In barely a few hours, Eduardo's body would become dust, ashes that I would spread according to his desire and that would be incorporated into the universe. I remained a few more instants alone, in front of the oven, in silence, peaceful, dazzled, lost in wonder.

When we left the cemetery, the sun was shining strongly in an almost cloudless sky. Mr Meyer drove me to Gisela's, in a small township close to the border with France, where I was expected for dinner. Since we arrived early, I had time to take a long walk in the grove surrounding the small residential area. In touch with nature, immersed in the beneficent peace of the forest that was enveloping me, I felt well, light, tenderly accompanied. I meditated and I spoke with Eduardo... I went back to the house as Gisela was starting to prepare the meal. While she was cooking, we chatted like two old friends. I had a special request for her: if possible, I wanted to go back home with a copy of the two videos taken on the day of Eduardo's AVD. Knowing she would not see any inconvenience in this, I had brought a USB key. Her assistant transferred onto it the films in question, audio-visual souvenirs converting my USB key into a very precious object.

After the delicious dinner we shared with her assistant and her secretary, Gisela drove me to the tramway station. It was there that our roads were parting. Once out of the vehicle, we fell into each other's arms to say goodbye. I reiterated the deep gratitude I felt for what she had done for my son. Thanks to her, he had been able to free himself from his suffering. Yes, this AVD was really what he wanted; it was the most beautiful thing that could happen. For this I would be eternally grateful to her. She retorted that it had "to happen like that in order to avoid a drama in Québec." Indeed, after we met in May, she knew what Eduardo had asked me to do if he did not get assisted suicide, and she knew I had the strength to bring his project to fruition even clandestinely.

We warmly hugged and kissed; then, she got into her car and rushed to her next meeting. After waiting for a few minutes, I boarded the tramway taking me back to Basel, happy with this last day on Swiss land.

At the hotel, my luggage was ready. The following day, I was catching a flight back to Canada... in a wheelchair!

At the End of His Struggle

Eduardo went to Switzerland to receive help in ending his life. If Eduardo's life had been respected, he would have died naturally on November 20, 2002. That is to say that if he had not been resuscitated, Eduardo could have died in peace and without pain. But doctors intervened and resuscitated him. Consequently, he suffered horribly during all the life that was imposed on him and had to resort to assisted suicide to free himself from his sufferings and reclaim his death.

Eduardo would never have had to commit suicide if doctors had respected his life. We need to be aware of that.

How many people end up, like Eduardo, in unsustainable situations because of medical intervention? Eduardo had the chance—if you can say that—to be able to formulate his request for help in dying. But how many persons are forced to endure the fate others have decided for them? In a society like ours, led by technology and protocols of all kinds, medical aid in dying must be offered in a much more supple manner than the one described in the law.

What hurts me is not so much that Eduardo died, but rather that he suffered during all those years. It is all those interminable years of painful and endless struggle that break my heart. That I had to look at him dying every day, this is what hurts me. Throughout Eduardo's liberation process, I constantly went back, in spite of myself, to the starting point—his resuscitation—and I relived, innumerable times, the calvary that has been his. If only we had let him die...

Eduardo was greatly disappointed by the fact that nobody wanted to listen to him. I must say that we had been chasing rainbows. Eduardo believed his story would interest everyone, and so did I. To be a victim and a survivor of a poorly effective and highly risky medical intervention, systematically performed without consent, was this not making him the ideal subject of an interview or an article? We had thus imagined ourselves being invited to a TV program to give a testimony or maybe becoming the topic of a news story. We even went as far as practicing our responses to hypothetical questions asked by an imaginary reporter. Wasted effort.

From the moment Eduardo asked me for assisted suicide, it was preferable not to attract attention to his story, in order to prevent anyone from interfering with his project. In spite of this, when our book came out in its French version, I could not help but send, to five CBC (Canadian Broadcasting Corporation) programs, a copy of the book accompanied by a letter of presentation. It was on my part a spontaneous gesture, an ignored risk, a desperate attempt (maybe?) to attract a journalist's interest and to give Eduardo the gift he deserved: to be heard.

However, this did not go very far, for I did not receive any response. Absolutely no answer. Given the circumstances, it was better this way. But to what could I attribute this silence? Had the book come at the wrong time? Were the journalists overloaded with work or concentrated on more important issues? Were the agendas already full? Why was this poignant account, so revealing on the realities and the consequences of CPR, being ignored? Was this survivor's testimony considered too unsettling, too threatening for the status quo? It was not the first time I was treated with indifference. In the course of the preceding year, I had contacted many people in management positions—in Eduardo's country of origin—and almost all my interventions had fallen on deaf ears. This new silence was not surprising to me. I knew what it meant: I was being told, once more, that my son was a collateral damage. What outrage! I considered that in the name of liberty, of integrity, of inviolability, of human dignity, this true story had to be known. At that moment a question rose in me that I am still asking myself: "This is CBC News, whatever happens," what does it really mean?

Now that Eduardo has liberated himself, that he can no longer be harmed in any way, I have free rein and I can scream my revolt in front of what is unacceptable, unjustifiable.

A little inner voice insisted I express myself with tact and delicacy, but I swiftly muted it, preferring a tone as biting as that of Eduardo, who said, "Doctors would have to live the same that I have lived in order to understand."He was right. What do they, doctors, imagine? That they are here "to save lives" at all costs? That they have the right to endanger people's well-being in applying aggressive protocols (in case it works) because they want to prevent them from dying? They would do better to come down from their pedestal and stop playing gods. A good bath of humility would not hurt them either. Doctors are not at the service of life but at the service of persons in need. Their main mission is to take care of their patients in an open and honest relationship, always seeking their greatest well-being. *Primum non nocere*.

After all I have lived with Eduardo, I cannot help making a parallel between medical aid in dying (MAID) and cardiopulmonary resuscitation (CPR), the latter being a good example of medical aid in suffering. Why so much resistance in the face of MAID and none in the face of CPR? Why so many conditions imposed on a suffering person who makes a decision for his/her own life? And why no safeguard measures concerning CPR, an intervention that is not chosen knowingly but performed systematically on many people according to pre-established protocols? For MAID, the informed consent must be strictly applied; for CPR, on the other hand, no consent is required and, moreover, do-not-resuscitate orders are sometimes disregarded. How informed is this decision (made by the medical authorities) to impose CPR on almost everyone who dies suddenly, presuming their consent? Why so much caution and consultation with MAID and so little questioning with CPR? Yet CPR consequences are as irreversible as those of MAID, not to mention that CPR is very costly in human suffering.

Eduardo's story is a golden testimony reminding us that every human being is untouchable, that death is part of life, that it belongs to each person and that it must be respected. As so many others, Eduardo was a victim of medical technology, a collateral damage of thoughtless human action, blinded by an incredible arrogance. And also a collateral damage of a medical practice that is suffering from a lack of truth. Is not being a collateral damage of an action plan systemized by health services something completely unacceptable, something reprehensible? Eduardo's extraordinary journey urges us to face reality and to question the legitimacy of cardiopulmonary resuscitation, an intervention that, undeniably, infringes upon the dignity of the person.

About CPR

Eduardo journeyed laboriously on painful paths, estranged from the destiny that was his; he went through unimaginable ordeals and endured what nobody would wish to have to face; he lived a life of constant suffering that nobody would ever want. At the end of his struggle, I do not have the right to stay silent. I have the responsibility to denounce the universal implementation of cardiopulmonary resuscitation (CPR), a situation that nothing can justify, neither medically nor ethically speaking.

Myth. It all started one day, at the beginning of the sixties, when some physicians-researchers succeeded in restarting the heart of a few patients by means of external cardiac massage. After the publication of their results, according to which 14 patients out of 20 had recovered completely, everybody got carried away. It is without considering the conditions in which these persons had been resuscitated (in the operating room, because of complications due to anesthesia) that the new technique was rapidly associated to mouth to mouth ventilation to create what we now know as CPR. It was believed that the means to save people from death had been found! Since then, enthusiasm has never faded out within the medical community. CPR started to be used—and is still persistently used—on all the people suffering a cardiac arrest, independently of their health status or of their personal circumstances. Cardiac arrest has been transformed into a treatable condition and, very rapidly, CPR has become a universal and incontestable procedure, the default procedure to adopt before any cardiac arrest. Right from the beginning of its use on a wide scale, the low success rate of CPR (less than 10%) and the severe brain damage it causes to the survivors were noticed, which, instead of calling into question the established intervention protocols, has rather been a motivation to pursue the clinical research in the field. The famous "chain of survival" has been invented and, with sensitization campaigns and well thought of slogans, the population has been encouraged to learn the CPR maneuvers, all of this in an effort to increase survival rates—which, actually, have not noticeably varied over decades. Quite perniciously, a real myth has been woven around cardiopulmonary resuscitation in such a way that a lot of people think that CPR works in most cases and that resuscitated people go back to the lives they had before the cardiac arrest. Everybody seems to be convinced that cardiac arrest is a health problem and that in applying CPR, lives are saved. Not only the media but also doctors, researchers, scientific societies and diverse official organizations have all contributed (and continue to do so) to this situation. Moreover, legislative bodies all over the world have followed suit. Here, in Québec, CPR intervention protocols are strongly protected—in fact even sanctioned—by some legal provisions, that is to say Article 13 of the Québec Civil Code, which allows intervening without consent in case of emergency, and Article 2 of the Charter of Rights and Freedoms, which guarantees the right to be rescued for every person whose life is in peril. Furthermore, CPR has been trivialized to such a point that its learning has become compulsory for high school students and soon will be for primary school pupils as well! Ignoring the poor results obtained with CPR, its proponents have taken steps to transmit the message that together we can—we must—save lives! And they have been successful. The CPR myth is everywhere present. But what exactly is the situation?

Reality. First of all, when speaking about CPR, we must know we are speaking of death. Because cardiac arrest is death. The signs and symptoms for the diagnosis of cardiac arrest are the same doctors have traditionally used to ascertain death. Cardiac arrest is not a disease, an electrical imbalance or a temporary failing of the heart; it is not some kind of pathology that can be cured. When the heart stops, the person passes away and it is the beginning of one's death process. When cardiac arrest occurs in an unexpected and sudden manner, it is called sudden death. While it is true that with the development of CPR, it has been agreed to consider cardiac arrest no longer as death but as an emergency life-threatening pathological event, this semantic manipulation of concepts changes nothing to the reality. Death is always death. And what we are trying to do with CPR is to counter death.

CPR, a set of maneuvers to reverse cardiac arrest, can be described as a "brutal attack," a violent and bloody attack on a person who has just died. The trauma inflicted to the whole body is major: broken ribs, broken teeth, injuries to the respiratory tract and to other internal organs (including the heart), pneumonias, hemorrhages and generalized shock. But the most serious lesion, the one that determines the patient's prognosis, is the devastating brain damage produced by CPR maneuvers. CPR is an intervention that fails in 70 to 98% of the cases; and when it succeeds (that is to say when a pulse is recovered), the person is admitted to the intensive care unit to receive advanced life support according to aggressive protocols—not devoid of unwanted side effects—that offer only a very thin hope of recuperation.

Results. Scientific articles on the subject speak of survival for out-of-hospital cardiac arrest. It is wrong to speak this way, since there cannot be survival from death. In 40 to 50% of the people who die suddenly, no resuscitation maneuvers are undertaken, as they are considered dead for too long. The observed survival is due to the fact that CPR is performed and that, afterward, at the end of a more or less long stay in the intensive care unit, some people end up not dying. In reality, one should speak of CPR survival. In fact, the survival rates being reported in studies and newspaper articles refer to the percentage of people surviving among those on whom CPR maneuvers were undertaken. What are the results? From all the people on whom resuscitation is attempted, the majority (70 to 75%) dies in the field or at the emergency room. Among those who recover a pulse and are subjected to life-sustaining measures, mortality is also very high, about 65 to 70%. The published results—manipulated from the start and calculated at very short term—vary a lot according to studies, hospitals and world regions; but globally, the average survival does not reach 8% for out-of-hospital cardiac arrests treated with CPR.

It should be stressed that all the people whose cardiac arrest occurs in certain circumstances (trauma, drowning, intoxication, hanging, electrocution, asphyxia) are excluded from the survival rates reported in the studies of out-of-hospital cardiac arrest, which focus on cardiac arrests of purely cardiac origin. Furthermore, many people are lost in the follow-up and are also excluded from the results. Which means that the real CPR survival rates are probably lower than those published.

Moreover, several factors diminish CPR survival chances, among others, absence of witness, non-shockable initial rhythm, no recovery of a pulse in the field (or late pulse recovery) and being at home at the time of the arrest, without forgetting pre-arrest existing pathologies, like cardiac or liver failure, diabetes, arterial hypertension, dyslipidemia, kidney or pulmonary disease, or metastasized cancer. Given the multiple factors in play, it is very difficult to make a prediction. However, some data clearly come out of the studies carried out up to now. We know, for example, that the prognosis remains very bleak (survival less than 2%) for most people who do not recover a pulse in the field and that the chances of survival do not exceed 0.5% for those people who meet the three following criteria: 1) the arrest is not witnessed by emergency team personnel; 2) no defibrillator shock is delivered; and 3) no pulse recovery in the field.

Let us take some examples rounding up the survival rate at 10%. Let us suppose that a person suffers a cardiac arrest in the presence of a witness. The survival chances are, theoretically, 10% with the intervention of emergency services, but will vary depending on the cardiac rhythm initially detected: if the person is found in ventricular fibrillation (shockable rhythm, present in only 20 to 25% of the cases), the survival chances can reach 30%; but if found in asystole (non-shockable rhythm), there is almost no chance of survival, between 1 and 2%. Let us imagine now a woman about 65 years old who is found unconscious, unresponsive and without a pulse by a passerby. The latter calls the emergency services and starts to give her CPR. What are the chances for this woman, after being resuscitated, to come out in a good state and with normal cerebral function? No more than 2%.

It is important to remember that even if ventricular fibrillation is associated with better survival chances, the resuscitation efforts on most people with this rhythm result in failure (about 70% mortality). Let us also say there is a sub-category of victims who are not declared dead in spite of the clinical signs of death persisting after 20 or 30 minutes of CPR but who are rather considered as being in "refractory cardiac arrest"! These persons are transported if possible to a specialized hospital where they are subjected to specific interventions intended to snatch them from death, an approach leading to few survivors, many of them in very bad state. What to say? This goes beyond comprehension!

Ultimately, in order to "save" the lives of only a few people, dozens of others must be "tortured": those who die sooner or later after the CPR maneuvers have begun and also those who survive CPR but remain in an unsustainable situation. What is the ethical ground for such a practice?

Prognosis. It is not enough to survive. One must survive well. A rather stunning fact: for a long time, doctors-researchers focused on the survival rates without worrying too much about the survivors' neurological state. Since this aspect has been taken into consideration, they strive to devise a useful prognostication tool. However, they have stressed the negative prognosis: they try to determine with 100% certainty which people have a negative prognosis, that is to say those who will progress toward death or serious neurological damage, the latter resulting in coma, vegetative state or severe disability. The consequences? Many victims are uselessly subjected to life-sustaining treatments for several days (because they do not meet the established criteria predicting a negative prognosis) and end up leaving the intensive care unit in a disastrous situation, worse than death.

By all accounts, doctors-researchers are on the wrong path. Firstly, because certainty does not exist, neither in medicine nor in life in general. Secondly, because considering only death and serious neurological damage as negative prognosis does not reflect the reality. There is a whole array of clinical situations, very painful and not at all desirable, that should be included in the negative prognosis and that people should be made aware of. And thirdly, because this is an attitude contrary to all ethics. It is unjustifiable to play with people's lives this way.

Why did not the doctors-researchers choose to focus on the positive prognosis? And since they want so much to be certain before acting, why not seek to identify with 100% certainty the people with a positive prognosis? Why not limit interventions to the people who have all the chances to survive well? This could save numerous victims from inhuman treatments.

Consequences. How are the CPR survivors doing? There are apparently some people who go back to their lives in a satisfactory way: they are those who are used in the publicity around CPR, exceptions who were lucky. About all the others nothing is said. Many are the doctors-researchers who affirm that most of the survivors are "neurologically intact," but this is false. They make this claim because they consider as such all those who are in categories 1 and 2 on the CPC (Cerebral Performance Categories) rating scale. Persons included in these categories may present either minor neurological or psychological deficiencies, like mild dysphasia, nonincapacitating hemiparesis or minor cranial nerve abnormalities; or a moderate disability, that is to say hemiplegia (paralysis of one half of the body), seizures, ataxia (problems with balance and coordination), dysarthria (speech difficulties), or also permanent alterations of the memory or other mental processes. Those are severe sequelae that considerably diminish the quality of life. Furthermore, fatigue, long-term cognitive deficits and emotional problems are frequent in all survivors, many of whom have to struggle to go back to work and re-establish a significant social life.

What about the survivors in categories 3 and 4 on the rating scale? If one believes the results of a great number of doctors-researchers, they represent between 20% and 30% of the survivors. This proportion, however, grows to 50% according to many other authors, which certainly better reflects the reality. Persons in category 3 are conscious but severely disabled: they cannot live alone and need help for everything; those in category 4 are in a vegetative state or in a coma. Collateral damage, like Eduardo, no one wants to talk about.

Moreover, CPR survivors are not the only ones suffering. For their life partners and their families, life is not the same anymore. They are overburdened by new responsibilities (care, supervision, support, etc.) toward their diminished relative, and are often faced with problems of depression, anxiety and post-traumatic stress.

We hear about community resources providing for the particular needs of the survivors. But what are they? There is an appalling lack of resources! Besides, is there really a will to help all these victims with neurological damage? In the last two years of Eduardo's life, we lost our home support. The person coming to help us 18 hours a week had found a better use of her time, and we had been unable to replace her. No social worker called or came home for a follow-up to check how we were doing. Since Eduardo was not costing anything to the system...

Benefit. The priority goal of any medical treatment is to benefit the patient. As moral agents, physicians must act as far as possible to preserve the health and to alleviate the suffering of their patients—not to cause it!—and this, always with respect for the person. They must thus offer their patients therapeutic options that will contribute to their well-being. To save life at all costs is not among physicians' prerogatives.

An appropriate medical intervention is one that offers a reasonable hope of amelioration without deleterious side effects and whose benefit/risks ratio is clearly favorable to the patient. If CPR offered 90% survival chances and did not produce the multiple medical problems and handicaps affecting the survivors, it could be considered appropriate. Even then, consent should be sought before performing it, since it is about interfering in a person's death process, a transcendent and intimate event.

The reality is such that neither from a medical nor an ethical point of view can CPR be objectively qualified as beneficent nor can its systematic use be justified. Despite this evidence, international recommendations in the matter of resuscitation are maintained, and doctors-researchers strive to reach a consensus on what should be considered as a satisfactory outcome. A consensus on such a personal question as quality of life?! Is it not evident that to benefit the patient, CPR should give them back their life as they knew it? To survive having lost the capacity to pursue one's life project or being totally dependent on others does not constitute a benefit for the patient. That is, however, what is awaiting a good part of the CPR survivors.

Given the distressing panorama offered by CPR, it is essential to provide each person with the pertinent information in order for one to be able to choose which risks are worth taking. Thus all citizens could make known their will to be resuscitated by means of their health card.

Emergency. Article 13 of Québec Civil Code stipulates, "Consent to medical care is not required in case of emergency if the life of the person is in danger or his integrity threatened and his consent cannot be obtained in due time." Okay. But cardiac arrest is not a potentially fatal acute condition. Death does not endanger one's life nor does it threatens one's integrity. It is the CPR maneuvers that do that, that plunge the person into a horrible situation extending the death process or eventually leading to severe and permanent bodily injuries.

Curiously, everybody seems to have overlooked paragraph 2 of Article 13 of the Civil Code: "**It [consent] is required, however**, where the care is unusual or has become useless or **where its consequences could be intolerable for the person**." (bold font mine) This is exactly the case for CPR. It follows that it should only be performed on persons who consent to such a procedure. Emergency certainly does not give the right to place someone in a situation worse than their natural death.

Besides, this emergency pretext in case of sudden death no longer holds water today. After more than 50 years of cardiopulmonary resuscitation and all kinds of studies, the question is extensively known as are the poor CPR results. What is urgently needed, on the other hand, is to tell the whole truth to the population.

Right to rescue. According to Article 2 of the Charter of Human Rights and Freedoms, "every human being whose life is in peril has a right to assistance." I must say it again: once death has occurred, life is no longer in peril. It has simply ended. To rescue someone in distress goes without saying, of course, for example, when the person is wounded, has an allergic reaction or is stuck somewhere, or when he/she is unconscious but alive. However, when someone has just died, they do not need to be rescued. And they do not need either to have their death profaned with impunity.

Let us not forget either that every person has the right to refuse to be rescued. The anticipated will of a person not to be resuscitated, which can be expressed in a personal document (ex: a letter, a medical bracelet or a wallet card), is valid everywhere and must be respected by everyone, without exception. It must however be easily accessible, otherwise one is resuscitated without consent!

How is it that CPR, an intervention so ineffective and so harmful, has become part of the compulsory first aid protocols and is as such protected by the law? I still don't get it.

I can understand that some people want to live at all costs, so let them be resuscitated. At their own risk! But, please, could we leave in peace all those who prefer to die a natural death?

Dignity. The right to life is inseparable from the inherent dignity of every human being, and from this dignity follow all the rights protected by the Charter of Human Rights and Freedoms. The objective to save lives cannot ignore this absolute and untouchable reality: the person in all his/her dignity.

Human dignity is a reality difficult to grasp. Yet dignity can be understood very quickly by being slightly or temporarily deprived of it. It is undeniable that the notions of freedom, autonomy, integrity and inviolability are inextricably tied to the dignity of the person.

There is affront to dignity when one loses the capacity to make fundamental personal choices. There is affront to dignity when one loses their freedom or the capacity to exercise their rights. There is affront to dignity when one loses the control of one's body or is mutilated because of some intervention. There is affront to dignity when one can no longer enjoy any intimacy or private life. There is affront to dignity when the life, and thus the death, of someone is not respected.

Careful! A person, whatever their circumstances may be, never loses their dignity. However, in situations where there is affront to dignity, the person is touched in what is most precious to them. Some people live very well in spite of several affronts to dignity, and others can absolutely not support it. Each person is unique and must be respected.

With the universal implementation of CPR, it has been decided that we would save lives. But at what price? To save lives in bringing back victims in any state? Striving to restart hearts with no regard for the persons? Is this saving lives? What about the inherent dignity of every human being? It is precisely because of this dignity that we do not have the right to interfere in someone's life! Is life worth living when dignity is compromised? This is for everyone to decide.

Consequently, no medical intervention having the potential to infringe upon human dignity—so no resuscitation—should be undertaken without the informed (really informed) and explicit consent of the person or of his/her legal representative.

End of life. The Québec law concerning end-of-life care, entered into force on December 10, 2015, considers the provision of end-of-life care in recognition of and respect for the rights and freedoms of the person and determines, among others, that "end-of-life patients must be treated, at all times, with understanding, compassion, courtesy and fairness, and with respect for their dignity, autonomy, needs and safety."

Unfortunately, many people dying or at the end of life are not treated with the respect due to them. I am thinking, of course, of people who die suddenly, like Eduardo, but also of those in agony on the site of a serious accident. What happens to these people? They are implicitly but surely excluded from what is called end of life—which has not been defined by the legislator—and they find themselves victims of an absurd therapeutic relentlessness, unfounded and disrespectful of their person.

Nonetheless, people who die suddenly are people at the end of life. It needs to be acknowledged. They have the right to die suddenly and to be respected in their end of life, to be respected in the death that belongs to them. I do not know anybody who would like to spend the last days of their lives in an intensive care unit. The law concerning end-of-life care should apply, without discrimination, to everyone at the end of life, and not only to those who are old and in the terminal stage of an incurable disease.

Information. We must tell things the way they are. People have the right to receive complete, truthful and unfiltered information about CPR, and doctors have the duty to provide them with it. In the era of modern communications, it is totally unacceptable to perpetuate the state of disinformation in which the population remains.

When people are told that survival chances might double if they give CPR, they must also be told what this means: that survival chances go, for example, from 2% to 4% or from 8% to 16% only. To encourage people to give CPR without telling them the serious damage caused by resuscitation is showing a lack of honesty. To make believe that with CPR we save lives without clearly specifying the possible results is deluding people. Not to explicitly speak of the painful situations in which survivors end up is hiding the truth. To lead the population in a "chain of survival" along and at the end of which a multitude of people suffer uselessly and without consent is showing a lack of integrity. To divulge only out of context fragments of information is failing an elementary deontological duty.

At present, most people greatly overestimate CPR effectiveness and nurture false hopes. But if they knew the whole story, how would they react? If they knew what to really expect, what would they choose?

The lack of information is blatant, as shown by the numerous conflictual situations happening every day in hospitals when someone is admitted in a comatose state after having been resuscitated. Besides being emotionally distressing for all the persons involved, they often give rise to difficult confrontations between the victim's relatives and the members of the healthcare team. The so-called CPR benefits have been insisted upon so much that it is understandable for the victim's family to expect excellent results and to insist on receiving a definite prognosis as soon as possible, which the intensive care physicians are unable to do. Obviously, the intensive care unit is not the ideal place to start an honest discussion about CPR consequences. In other hospital services or in long-term care facilities, it is not surprising either that seriously ill patients, firmly believing CPR to be a good solution, expect to receive it and even go so far as to demand it in spite of their poor health condition. They have been convinced that CPR saves lives, so why not theirs! They cannot understand why they are told at the last moment that CPR is not medically appropriate in their case. On one side, the directive issued in many health institutions is to perform CPR in all cases unless there is an explicit counter-order; and on the other, the physician's clinical judgement sometimes contradicts this directive, which is the source of great confusion. These situations too are very unpleasant and sometimes lead to absurd legal proceedings that only complicate things. Doctors should not wait to be considering a do-not-resuscitate order to openly communicate and have frank discussions with their patients about CPR; they should do so as soon as they receive them into their care. In fact, it is for the population in its entirety that the medical authorities should be raising awareness about CPR realities, as it is known that sudden death happens mostly at home. It is also known that everywhere, in private and nursing homes, in the streets, the train stations, the airports, the shopping malls, etc. live and move around people with diverse pathologies that diminish their chances of surviving CPR. They have the right to know. Each person, hospitalized or not, must be able to refuse to be resuscitated in case of sudden death and thus needs to be correctly informed.

Another important thing: the science of resuscitation is a vast field of clinical experimentation to which different groups of doctors-researchers everywhere in the world participate assiduously. All committed to the same task, to advance the science of resuscitation, they collaborate regularly to update the guidelines regarding CPR. What is the value of the evidence on which these guidelines rest? In terms of the quality of the evidence provided, scientific works are classified in five levels of evidence, the strongest being randomized controlled trials and the weakest expert opinions. People should know that most of the clinical studies are tainted by bias of all kinds, which render their conclusions more or less reliable. What's more, when clinical trials are financed by pharmaceutical companies (and many are), we must be particularly cautious. Actually, the famous "scientific evidence" does not always provide evidence, thus one must read the scientific literature with a critical sense. Regarding CPR, the majority of the recommendations issued are supported by works with a low or very low level of evidence. That is to say that the recommendations for resuscitation rest mostly on speculations without valid scientific grounds. The truth is there is no evidence justifying the universal implementation of CPR.

Then, why such a well-structured system to "save life"? It must be concluded that some interests are very well served by this deployment of technology and heroic efforts, interests that, I am afraid, have nothing to do with people's well-being.

It should be noted that "technological progress" and CPR have changed the perspectives in the medical world. At the end of the sixties, a new definition of death was invented (brain death) to allow the removal of organs in patients judged unsalvageable (because of severely impaired consciousness) who were relying on technology for their survival. Since then, there has been a lot of water under the bridge and all means are good to ward off death. It is now current practice to use people who die suddenly in enrolling them in clinical studies—with anticipated consent!—in order to increase our knowledge about cardiac arrest, resuscitation and advanced life support techniques. At the same time, there is also another practice, already well established in many countries: going back to cardiac arrest criteria for death diagnosis and deciding, after 20 or 30 minutes of CPR without pulse recovery, to treat the victim as a potential organ and tissue donor—which is done with presumed consent! We are thus disposing of the body in a spirit of productivity, as if the body no longer belonged to the person, as if it was only a collection of "detachable pieces" from which we have the right to benefit to serve the interests of someone else. This is medical utilitarianism. The worst is how easily it is justified, in claiming objectives considered very laudable and playing with people's emotions. Medico-scientific progress is leading the way, it seems to me, and is constantly feeding the absurd desire to vanquish death! So there it is, a great many people are resuscitated—people who are going to die anyway, but after hours or days of agony—only to "save" a few among whom many are condemned to a poor quality survival. Personally, I do not wish to serve as a guinea pig to all these scientists with rather questionable ethics. And you?

Questioning. It can only come from the acceptance of reality: things not as we imagine them but as they are. Death being part of life, wanting to fight it makes no sense. We have no other choice but to accept our finitude and all the uncertainties that are part and parcel of human life. To live well, to live as well as possible, one simply needs to take care of oneself. This is what true prevention is. Yes, because life is precious, it is not about fighting death but about taking care of oneself all along the way. And then, when death comes, knowing how to bow down, let go and enter this sacred unknown that liberates from all ailments...

Besides, do not doctors commit themselves to take care of their patients? to look after their patients' well-being with respect for their dignity? Thus they should be the first ones to question the universal and indiscriminate implementation of CPR, an aberrant plan of action generating painful and artificial agonies, cold and prolonged deaths, and ruined lives. In 2019, I got in touch with diverse health and ethics organizations with the aim to draw their attention on the ravages caused by CPR, but my attempts went nowhere. I had nourished the hope that among all the persons contacted, at least one of them would let himself/herself be challenged by the serious and sincere testimony coming not only from a survivor's mother but also from a former member of the medical profession. But this didn't happen. I have been for all practical purposes ignored. Once again, the same outrageous and inadmissible message: Eduardo was a collateral damage. I was sadly realizing how much one can be narrow-minded and how easily one can choose to comfortably assume a position that is disembodied, irresponsible and devoid of sensitivity.

Yet, from the results achieved with CPR, logical and honest conclusions should be drawn: CPR only saves lives in exceptional conditions and makes a multitude of innocent victims, which justifies modifying the intervention protocols in emergency medicine. If we ceased blindly resuscitating everyone, numerous undesired catastrophic situations could be avoided. Sticking to the preconceived idea that sudden death is unacceptable and insisting in finding ways to increase the number of survivors at all costs instead of facing reality is neither scientific nor is it respectful of human life. It is the well-being of each person that matters, not the survival rate in the population. Besides, mortality is always 100% since we will all die one day, in one manner or another. It seems to me that respecting someone's death is an ineluctable moral imperative, more so when one is a physician.

Wanting to explain sudden death simply by the obstruction of coronary arteries, the presence of a cardiomyopathy or the occurrence of a malignant arrhythmia and fixing the "problem" by resuscitating the person is showing a very reductionist view. The heart that stops is inside a body that belongs to a person who evolves in a certain milieu and who has a very singular life story, a journey distinct from that of everyone else. We should not lose sight of the fact that the profound reasons of death are anchored in the person's experience. But now in medicine, as in other domains, we seem willing to get around reality and ignore the mystery residing at the heart of each person. Provided with a more and more sophisticated technology and motivated by hubris, we have decided to take charge of life imperfections. In addition to fixing objectives, juggling with concepts and establishing protocols, we like to dissect things, to decompose them and to simplify them in order to better manipulate and control them, without taking into account the complexity of human life, forgetting that any event (including sudden death) occurs in a very personal context we cannot ignore. I explained all this to Eduardo, one day, during one of our many conversations about his resuscitation. Here is his commentary, "Ah! So doctors use only their left hemisphere?!" To the point. It would be nice to find a way to stimulate the doctors' and researchers' right hemisphere; maybe this way a real questioning could begin? And if, as Eduardo mentioned to me, money was taken away from doctors for each mutilated resuscitated person? Then, I think things would rapidly take a different turn.

Finally, the universal implementation of CPR is without a doubt the most shocking manifestation of the categorical rejection of death. In considering death as a failure—and perhaps also in exploiting the fear of death present in everyone—we have come to impose intervention protocols meeting the arbitrary objectives we have fixed, objectives at the population level that do not consider the well-being of each individual. How is it that such protocols, encroaching upon the freedoms and fundamental rights of the person, are tolerated and never questioned??!! Would the medical establishment be enjoying, without our knowledge, a special exemption in regard to the Charter of Rights and Freedoms allowing it to impose protocols that violate people's physical, psychological and spiritual integrity?

It must be said out loud and repeated: death, in any way that it occurs, is a personal matter. It is as sacred as life itself. We have no right to manage it with collective plans of action. Are not the primacy of the person over the collectivity and the safeguard of his/her dignity as a human being above any state or societal ambition? Let us be aware that a society's well-being can only be forged from the well-being of each of its members.

No matter how noble the intentions at the root of a project are, the interests of medical research must never prevail over people's well-being and respect for their dignity. To counter this very real threat and escape the abominable drifts that risk carrying us astray—that are already carrying us astray!—, I think everybody should take a step backward and remember the Nuremberg trial.

The Last Words

After so much suffering, Eduardo could reclaim his death.

Such happiness...

But, after so much suffering, will my bruised being hurt forever?

Eduardo has set himself free.

Such joy...

Our odyssey is over. In walking by Eduardo's side, I went to the end of myself.

I am proud of what we have achieved together.

Today, Eduardo is gone; I am alone, but I can still hope that his life testimony will propagate and touch future generations.

From this hope, I will nourish myself, I will live and continue my journey.

WE HAD NO RIGHT TO
ROB HIM OF HIS DEATH!

Post Scriptum

As for *Why was I resuscitated?*, this book is an authentic life testimony. In taking another look at cardiopulmonary resuscitation in the second last chapter—for obvious reasons—I wanted to push the reflection a little further. Because of the nature of this work, I have nonetheless restrained myself from overloading it with bibliographical references.

I have written this book plunged in Eduardo's grief, for it couldn't be otherwise. My state of mind has not allowed me to handle the pen with the ease I would have liked to display. I am sorry about it. I think, however, that Eduardo would be—that he is—satisfied with my work. In spite of everything, I have been able, in this little narrative strewn with imperfections, to tell as faithfully as possible the end of his story. Moved, I rejoice in this precious testimony.

Acknowledgement

In all my solitude, I have been blessed with the help of a few supportive persons to whom I wish to express my gratitude.

Thanks to Ana for her generous contribution: she dedicated part of her precious time in revising the whole manuscript with the attentiveness I know to be hers.

Thanks to Manon for her close collaboration: she went above and beyond the reader task I had given her and made very pertinent observations.

Thanks particularly to Martine for her faithful presence and her inestimable support: the multiple exchanges we had together sustained me all along my writing work.

To the three of them, thanks from the bottom of my heart.

About the author

Born in Saint-Joseph de Beauce, a small town in the province of Québec, Canada, Anne Beaudoin studied in several different fields before entering the Faculty of Medicine of the University of Sherbrooke, where she obtained her degree of *Medicinae Doctor, M.D.* in 1990. She completed her training in pediatrics at the Reina Sofía University Hospital of Córdoba, Spain. Retired for many years, she considers herself lucky to have been able to earn a living interacting passionately with the children and families she has attended to. From the summer of 2008 to September 5, 2019, she devoted herself exclusively to the care and support of her son Eduardo. She lives in Québec City.

www.ingramcontent.com/pod-product-compliance
Ingram Content Group UK Ltd.
Pitfield, Milton Keynes, MK11 3LW, UK
UKHW021932200726
13853UKWH00010B/357